SO-BXE-966

Technology:
The Interface to Nursing
Educational Informatics

Guest Editor

Elizabeth E. Weiner, PhD, RN-BC, FAAN

NURSING CLINICS
OF NORTH AMERICA

www.nursing.theclinics.com

Consulting Editor
Suzanne S. Prevost, RN, PhD, COI

December 2008 • Volume 43 • Number 4

SAUNDERS an imprint of ELSEVIER, Inc.

W.B. SAUNDERS COMPANY

A Division of Elsevier Inc.

1600 John F. Kennedy Blvd., Suite 1800 • Philadelphia, PA 19103-2899

http://www.theclinics.com

NURSING CLINICS OF NORTH AMERICA Volume 43, Number 4
December 2008 ISSN 0029-6465, ISBN-13: 978-1-4160-6325-4, ISBN-10: 1-4160-6325-0

Editor: Katie Hartner

Nursing Clinics of North America (ISSN 0029-6465) is published quarterly by Elsevier Inc., 360 Park Avenue South, New York, NY 10010-1710. Months of issue are March, June, September, and December. Business and Editorial Offices: 1600 John F. Kennedy Blvd., Suite 1800, Philadelphia, PA 19103-2899. Customer Service Office: 6277 Sea Harbor Drive, Orlando, FL 32887-4800. Periodicals postage paid at New York, NY and additional mailing offices. Subscription price per year is, $133.00 (US individuals), $273.00 (US institutions), $228.00 (international individuals), $334.00 (international institutions), $184.00 (Canadian individuals), $334.00 (Canadian institutions), $70.00 (US students), and $115.00 (international students). To receive student/resident rate, orders must be accompanied by name of affiliated institution, date of term, and the signature of program/ residency coordinator on institution letterhead. Orders will be billed at individual rate until proof of status is received. Foreign air speed delivery is included in all *Clinics* subscription prices. All prices are subject to change without notice. **POSTMASTER:** Send address changes to *Nursing Clinics*, Elsevier Periodicals Customer Service, 11830 Westline Industrial Drive, St. Louis, MO 63146. **Customer Service: 1-800-654-2452 (US). From outside the United States, call 1-314-453-7041. Fax: 1-314-453-5170. E-mail: JournalsCustomerService-usa@elsevier.com** (for print support) and **JournalsOnlineSupport-usa@elsevier.com** (for online support).

Nursing Clinics of North America is covered in *EMBASE/Excerpta Medica, MEDLINE/PubMed (Index Medicus), Social Sciences Citation Index, Current Contents, ASCA, Cumulative Index to Nursing, RNdex Top 100,* and Allied Health Literature and International Nursing Index (INI).

Printed in the United States of America.

Contributors

CONSULTING EDITOR

SUZANNE S. PREVOST, RN, PhD, COI
Associate Dean, Practice and Community Engagement, University of Kentucky, Lexington, Kentucky

GUEST EDITOR

ELIZABETH E. WEINER, PhD, RN-BC, FAAN
Professor in Nursing and Senior Associate Dean for Informatics, School of Nursing; and Professor in Biomedical Informatics, School of Medicine, Vanderbilt University, Nashville, Tennessee

AUTHORS

JAMIE E. ADAM, MSN, RN, FNP, NP-C
Assistant Professor, School of Nursing, Middle Tennessee State University; and Family Nurse Practitioner, Primary Care & Hope Clinic, Murfreesboro, Tennessee

SHIRLEY W. CANTRELL, PhD, RN
Associate Professor of Nursing, School of Nursing, Middle Tennessee State University, Murfreesboro, Tennessee

CHRISTINE R. CURRAN, PhD, RN, CNA
Associate Chief Nursing Officer, UMass Memorial Medical Center University Campus, Worcester, Massachusetts; Former Associate Professor of Clinical Nursing, The Ohio State University College of Nursing, Columbus, Ohio

JUDITH A. EFFKEN, PhD, RN, FACMI, FAAN
Professor, The University of Arizona College of Nursing, Tucson, Arizona

CAROLE A. GASSERT, RN, PhD, FACMI, FAAN
Associate Professor Emerita of Nursing, University of Utah, College of Nursing, Salt Lake City, Utah

JEFFRY S. GORDON, PhD
Professor of Informatics, School of Nursing, Vanderbilt University, Nashville, Tennessee

MARY Z. MAYS, PhD
Research Associate Professor and Co-Director, Office of Transformational Technologies and Organizations, College of Nursing & Healthcare Innovation, Arizona State University, Phoenix, Arizona

MARILYN R. McFARLAND, PhD, RN, FNP-BC, CTN
Associate Professor of Nursing, School of Nursing, University of Michigan, Flint, Michigan

LEIGH ANN McINNIS, PhD, FNP-BC
Associate Professor, School of Nursing, Middle Tennessee State University, Murfreesboro, Tennessee

RENEE P. McLEOD, DNSc, APRN, BC, CPNP
Clinical Professor and Co-Director, Office of Transformational Technologies and Organizations, College of Nursing & Healthcare Innovation, Arizona State University, Phoenix, Arizona

RYAN McNEW, AAS, CNE
Senior LAN Manager, School of Nursing, Vanderbilt University, Nashville, Tennessee

SANDRA J. MIXER, PhD, RN
Assistant Professor of Nursing, College of Nursing, University of Tennessee, Knoxville, Tennessee

PATRICIA O'LEARY, DSN, RN, COI
Associate Professor of Nursing, School of Nursing, Middle Tennessee State University, Murfreesboro, Tennessee

MARIA OVERSTREET, PhD(C), RN, CCNS
Assistant Professor of Nursing, Vanderbilt School of Nursing, Nashville, Tennessee

PATRICIA A. TRANGENSTEIN, PhD, RN-BC
Professor in Nursing Informatics and Specialty Director Nursing Informatics Program, Vanderbilt University, School of Nursing, Nashville, Tennessee

KAREN S. WARD, PhD, RN, COI
Professor of Nursing and Associate Director Online Programs, School of Nursing, Middle Tennessee State University, Murfreesboro, Tennessee

ELIZABETH E. WEINER, PhD, RN-BC, FAAN
Professor in Nursing and Senior Associate Dean for Informatics, School of Nursing; and Professor in Biomedical Informatics, School of Medicine, Vanderbilt University, Nashville, Tennessee

Contents

This article provides an overview of the challenges and strategies faced by educational administrators in planning, delivering, and evaluating technology services to today's nursing students and faculty. Academic technology uses, examples, and support suggestions are provided so that educational administrators can effectively choose appropriate technologies geared to meet their educational objectives. The challenge comes with deciding the intended educational outcomes, and designing the appropriate educational milieu. Administrators are reminded to look to central administration to coordinate and participate in technology planning.

Health care information technology has the potential to achieve clinical transformation. Nursing students and faculty must be able to use these tools effectively to use data and knowledge in their practice. This article describes informatics competencies for four levels of nurses (beginning nurses, experienced nurses, informatics specialists, and informatics innovators). Recent activities to include informatics competencies in program outcomes are also described in relation to the clinical nurse leader, doctorate of nursing practice, and baccalaureate essentials documents.

Faculty members have a critical role in deciding the content that is taught to their nursing students. They must grasp the importance of using technology to facilitate learning and knowledge of informatics concepts and skills. This article describes a successful faculty development program that was aimed at upgrading the technology and informatics skills of the faculty while at the same time developing and threading informatics skills across the baccalaureate nursing curriculum.

In an ever-increasing hectic and mobile society, Web-based instructional tools can enhance and supplement student learning and improve communication and collaboration among participants, give rapid feedback on one's progress, and address diverse ways of learning. Web-based formats offer distinct advantages by allowing the learner to view course materials when they choose, from any Internet connection, and as often as they want. The challenge for nurse educators is to assimilate the knowledge and expertise to understand and appropriately use these tools. A variety of Web-based instructional tools are described in this article. As nurse educators increase their awareness of these potential adjuncts they can select appropriate applications that are supported by their institution to construct their own "toolkit."

The nursing and nursing faculty shortages have created a greater need for effective online learning strategies. Today's learners require the flexibility offered by online learning, but only when well grounded in sound teaching-learning principles. This article describes strategies for online learning designed to keep the needs of today's learners in mind. These strategies are focused on the resolution of technology problems as well as the learning process.

This article describes the environmental factors that have contributed to the recent rapid growth of nursing doctoral education at a distance. Early and recent efforts to deliver distance doctoral education are discussed, using The University of Arizona College of Nursing experience as the key exemplar. The Community of Inquiry model is introduced as an appropriate model for doctoral education and then used as a framework to evaluate the current state of the art in distance doctoral nursing education. Successes and challenges in delivering doctoral education from a distance are described.

Cultural diversity must be taken seriously by both faculty and students, and requires action by both parties for successful integration into online learning. Limited diversity in the nursing workforce or student population creates a need for learning cultural competence. Online transcultural nursing courses meet this learning need and provide opportunities for a variety of students and faculty participation from around the world. Successful online learning experiences can contribute to the provision of culturally competent nursing care.

Visual Literacy in the Online Environment

Sandra J. Mixer, Marilyn R. McFarland, and Leigh Ann McInnis

Visual literacy combines words and graphics to enhance learning. Students are immersed in digital literacy and multimodal learning; therefore, it is important for educators to embrace visual literacy and strike out beyond printed text, PowerPoint slides, and discussion boards. This article describes the use of visual literacy as a tool to enhance student learning. An example demonstrating the application of visual literacy to teach transcultural nursing in an online environment is provided. The Web site containing a copy of the visual literacy teaching tool is also available to readers.

Back to the Future: Personal Digital Assistants in Nursing Education

Renee P. McLeod and Mary Z. Mays

This article provides an overview of the current state of the art for incorporating personal digital assistants (PDAs) into nursing education. The development of PDA technology and the lessons learned by educators integrating PDA technology into nursing curricula are described. The current cycle of PDA evolution is discussed and contrasted with a proposed model for maximizing the impact of PDAs on technological innovation in nursing education and practice.

The Use of Simulation Technology in the Education of Nursing Students

Maria Overstreet

This article provides a broad overview of simulation use in nursing education. An example of a simulation experience focusing on the development and debriefing of a medication safety exercise is presented based on a theoretic approach. Questions for future consideration by nursing educators and researchers are also presented with the ultimate goal of producing safer patient care and more deliberate reflecting practitioners.

Developing the Online Survey

Jeffry S. Gordon and Ryan McNew

Institutions of higher education are now using Internet-based technology tools to conduct surveys for data collection. Research shows that the type and quality of responses one receives with online surveys are comparable with what one receives in paper-based surveys. Data collection can take place on Web-based surveys, e-mail–based surveys, and personal digital assistants/Smartphone devices. Web surveys can be subscription templates, software packages installed on one's own server, or created from scratch using Web programming development tools. All of these approaches have their advantages and disadvantages. The survey owner must make informed decisions as to the right technology to implement. The correct choice can save hours of work in sorting, organizing, and analyzing data.

THE CLINICS ARE NOW AVAILABLE ONLINE!
Access your subscription at:
www.theclinics.com

Preface

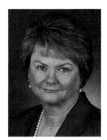

Elizabeth E. Weiner, PhD, RN-BC, FAAN
Guest Editor

Evidence surrounds us that technology is changing rapidly and affects us all in our daily lives. For example, most of us can hardly remember a world without cell phones. Today it is not uncommon to watch people multitasking in all walks of life while scrolling and texting on their Blackberries. Electronic mail seems to hold us hostage!

Nursing education is no different. I developed simulations in the early 80s, long before there were any high-fidelity simulators. We created a successful labor and delivery simulation on a 12-inch videodisc that allowed for either 30 minutes of video on each side of the disc or 24,000 individual frames. The result was that after we programmed a connecting computer, students could actually see the results of their decisions without threat to or interaction with a live patient. I have since framed that 12-inch videodisc in my office, and many who see it think it is a platinum record (for after all Vanderbilt is in Nashville, TN, the music city!). They have no historical framework for a 12-inch videodisc. I also developed an interactive tour of the Sigma Theta Tau International Virginia Henderson Library back in 1994, which we put onto a CD. One of those was buried in a time capsule at Headquarters to be opened sometime in the future. We had to laugh when we began to guess what people in the future might think was actually on that CD, because we expect they will not be able to play it. At least they could still use it to play Frisbee!

For all our frustration in trying to stay current with technology, we also realize that it holds the key to our ability to embrace nursing knowledge. It is only through technology that we stand the chance of organizing all of our data into information, information into knowledge, and thus use that knowledge to demonstrate wisdom. Our human brains do not themselves possess the ability to store and process such multitudes of data, nor do we have the ability to pass that process along to others as easily as the computer programs we create. It is imperative then that we master the technology tools to harness them into the knowledge-building activities that we need for the domain of nursing.

Nursing educators have been at the forefront of teaching technology skills to students, faculty, and staff, but have just begun to realize the potential of informatics use. Let me remind you that the word technology is not interchangeable with informatics. Technology is a tool that we use to assist us in the transition of data to information to knowledge to wisdom (which is informatics, and in our case, given that the domain is

Nurs Clin N Am 43 (2008) ix–x
doi:10.1016/j.cnur.2008.06.012
0029-6465/08/$ – see front matter

nursing, is called nursing informatics). Isn't there an intelligence that we faculty possess when we methodically design our nursing curriculum so that it is appropriately leveled and when completed meets our terminal objectives? How are we using technology to help us guide and gauge our students' progress? How do we know when students expand their critical thinking skills? Is there a way to integrate this growth from the simulated setting into the clinical setting? Isn't there a way to create a "student dashboard" so that students and faculty can actually see such progress? This is an example of nursing educational informatics.

We are in an era of designing our technology tools to better enable these educational informatics transactions. This edition of *Nursing Clinics of North America* does not present the end products of such a transition, but rather a delineation of technology tools that when used properly in the educational arena will start us on our productive way. Stay tuned for a later edition that might present such advanced examples of informatics use! In the meantime, enjoy this issue, which serves to help you better understand the technology tools that serve as an interface to the effective use of nursing educational informatics. My thanks are extended to all the busy authors who saw the value and potential of sharing their expertise with you so that together we can make a difference in educational informatics.

Elizabeth E. Weiner, PhD, RN-BC, FAAN
Vanderbilt University School of Nursing
461 21st Avenue South
Nashville, TN 37240, USA

E-mail address:
betsy.weiner@Vanderbilt.Edu (E.E. Weiner)

Supporting the Integration of Technology into Contemporary Nursing Education

Elizabeth E. Weiner, PhD, RN-BC, FAAN[a,b,*]

KEYWORDS

• Nursing education • Distance education
• Educational technology • Electronic learning
• Online education • Online learning

Supporting the nursing educational milieu of today is no longer a simple task of ensuring that the classroom is equipped with technology. The classroom itself has taken on such a virtual identity that the parameters of technology morph with the needs of the teachers and learners. While this situation allows for a multitude of choices and creativity in the design of educational activities, it has created a complex system of technology support that challenges even the best financed and experienced institutions. Furthermore, nurse educators and administrators must be flexible and responsive with effective and innovative solutions to complex market demands.[1]

What technology should be supported in nursing education? When should support shift to newer emerging technologies? How many people are required to provide needed support functions? What sort of budget is required to provide adequate support for faculty, staff, and students? What support should students expect if they operate primarily in a "distance" learning environment? All of these are critical questions for those educational administrators who need to adequately envision and plan for contemporary teaching and learning needs. Faculty members need to know what to expect when embarking on the transformation of their classrooms, and students need to know what to expect as far as reasonable support for their tuition dollars.

[a] Vanderbilt University, School of Nursing, 461 21st Avenue South, Nashville, TN 37240-2549, USA
[b] Vanderbilt University, School of Medicine, 2209 Garland Avenue, Nashville, TN 37232-8340, USA
* Vanderbilt University, School of Nursing, 461 21st Avenue South, Nashville, TN 37240-2549.
E-mail address: betsy.weiner@vanderbilt.edu

Nurs Clin N Am 43 (2008) 497–506
doi:10.1016/j.cnur.2008.06.002   nursing.theclinics.com
0029-6465/08/$ – see front matter © 2008 Elsevier Inc. All rights reserved.

This article provides an overview of the challenges of supporting technology in nursing education, and provides a scalable technology support model depending on the types of educational activities included in the curriculum. In addition, an overview of the accompanying articles in this issue is presented to provide a comprehensive picture of technology use in nursing education.

TRENDS IN HIGHER EDUCATION

For the first time, network security has become the number one concern for chief information officers in higher education.[2] This should come as no surprise to consumers who have watched the nightly news to frequently find stories related to identify theft, social security numbers lost, and threats to personal health data. Before this time, higher education has not seen security as an overwhelming matter of concern although it had previously made the top 10 EDUCAUSE list of concerns.[2] While educational administrators have always been concerned about student rights as related to FERPA (Family Educational Rights and Privacy Act), the academic health science centers are also having to contend with HIPAA (the Health Insurance Portability and Accountability Act). A security breach into a federal dataset has long-reaching implications, and it is important for the end users to practice proper network security in their day-to-day data management. Since 2003, the top three issues in terms of strategic importance to higher education have been administrative information technology (IT) systems, funding IT, and security.[2] The 2008 list of top 10 IT issues includes (1) security; (2) administrative IT systems; (3) funding IT; (4) infrastructure; (5) identity/access management; (6) disaster recovery; (7) governance, organization, leadership; (8) change management; (9) e-learning; and (10) staffing/human resource (HR) management/training.[2] Keep in mind that these results are from the overarching views of chief information officers, and are not necessarily the same views that the various colleges, schools, and departments might select. Faculty development is not on the list, but judging from recent nursing conferences is of grave concern to nursing in higher education.

Our nursing programs exist within larger systems that typically provide the IT infrastructure for all its academic units. As a result, some choices or priorities have already been set. (Note that this is why campus leadership in IT issues is so important.) For example, your campus may have already selected Blackboard as its course-based management system, so that your distributed support will center on faculty and staff development issues, student orientation, and providing local account support for access. Funding the purchase of additional servers or maintenance agreements becomes the responsibility of central administration.

Relying on central administration, however, can also have its negative impact. Their priorities may not be your priorities, such as a faculty database, or database of clinical placement facilities. Sometimes these applications must be developed at the local school level, keeping in mind that later there may be issues and problems related to systems integration. A decision will need to be made as to the relative risk of making the expenditures needed in hardware, software, and personnel for development and maintenance of the application. There is also the outside chance that if you have the need for such a software application, others may too, thus opening the possibility of selling or leasing the product for outside revenue.

Funding IT is always a challenge. While both hardware and software costs have been decreasing, bulk purchases continue to make up a large percentage of the budget. We have our hardware on a 3-year rotation cycle, and rotate the older machines out to our nurse-managed clinic sites whose electronic health record needs are not as robust as some of our research and simulation needs. This process actually gets about 3 to 4 more years from the computers, and politically satisfies their budget that never seems to be adequate because of the nonpayer mix of their clientele.

We have not typically provided both desktop and laptop computers for our faculty. Because of our increasingly mobile faculty environment, and along with the fact that so many of our programs are being taught as distance programs, for the first time we have split our hardware purchases so that half will be desktop machines and the other half laptops. We do not currently purchase cell phones or personal digital assistants (PDAs) for faculty use, except for those provided for via grants.

EMERGING TECHNOLOGIES FOR LEARNING

Unfortunately, while network security risks are at their greatest, the need for more social networking and communities is increasing at an exponential rate! Educational administrators are forced to make decisions that balance these two ends of the spectrum. As Skiba[3] describes, digital natives tend to communicate in the moment using instant messaging (IM), text messaging, blogging, expressing themselves on social networking sites, and now sending tweets. A tweet is a posting of 140 characters or less using an online application called Twitter, which is defined by Wikipedia as "a free social networking and microblogging service that allows users to send updates (tweets) to the Twitter Web site, via short message service, instant messaging, or a third-party application such as Twitterrific or Facebook."[4] Maag[5] provides a comprehensive discussion about the potential use of blogs in nursing education. She notes that Web logs, also known as "blogs," are an emerging writing tool that are easy to use, are Internet-based, and can enhance health professionals' writing, communication, collaboration, reading, and information-gathering skills. She further points out that a nursing school blog might motivate students to post their artwork, creative musings, and responses to case studies authored by instructors.[5]

Any technology tool that promotes critical thinking, analysis, and synthesis of information is worthy of careful consideration by faculty. WebQuests provide an additional example of just such a tool. As inquiry-oriented, engaging, and student-centered activities, WebQuests promote high-level thinking and problem-solving skills.[6] Using WebQuests, students construct their knowledge through guided inquiry-oriented activities that are heavily reliant on Internet resources. These activities can be either short (less than 1 week) or long term (1 to 4 weeks). As Lahaie[7] points out, "WebQuests have invigorated the K-12 educational sector around the globe, but there is sparse evidence in the literature about their use at the university levels." However, WebQuests are congruent with cognitive activities used in nursing education.

Today's health professions' educational programs have a unique mix of students from the Baby Boom Generation (born 1943 to 1960), Generation X (born 1961 to 1981), and Millennial, or Net, Generation (born 1982 to 2000), who demonstrate unique generational differences in the use of the Internet.[6] Unfortunately, in nursing education, we must try to address this broad range. Most of the aging faculty are from the Baby Boom Generation, and have to actively learn about how these new technologies can be used. At the same time, mobile devices and pervasive wireless networks are redefining the ways in which we live, work, play, and learn, because they provide ubiquitous access to digital tools and 24/7 access in popular and widely used portable forms.[8]

Prensky[9] notes that the most successful technology integration projects for learning activities have arisen when faculty have partnered with their students, who are eager to teach them. Students are "clamoring for these technologies to be used as part of their education, in part because they are things that the students have already mastered and use in their daily lives, and in part because they realize just how useful they can be."

Skiba[10] looked over articles in technology magazines and skimmed blogs of 2007 to highlight three significant trends that have implications for higher education and health care in 2008 and beyond. The first was touchscreens, as demonstrated by Apple's iPhone and representative of opening the door to many applications in a more user-friendly environment. The second trend was the rise in the social networking phenomenon, and the third trend was gaming. All three of these trends support the virtual reality revolution, which has the potential as a technology to change nursing education by bridging the education gap between knowledge and application.[11]

A discussion about emerging technologies would not be complete without the mention of the increased use of cell phones for campus alerts. While not directly a learning technology, this method of communication has been increasingly important recently as a result of a rise in campus violence. The shooting deaths of both students and faculty at Virginia Tech in 2007 directly resulted in many campuses investing or building campus alert systems that took advantage of the services of the various carriers to alert users of crises that could not be otherwise be directly communicated.

TECHNOLOGY SUPPORT MODELS

So how does an informed nursing education administrator decide just what to support? Rather than letting technology drive education, education should provocatively make clear what education needs from technology.[12] It is not enough to advertise that your school uses the "newest" form of technology, especially if you have the technology for the sake of having it rather than using it in a meaningful way. This sort of purchase may in fact "backfire," causing students to wonder why their precious funds were used to purchase something that was never appropriately used. The technological choices should be a response to stated needs of education and not a stimulus to change for its own sake.[12]

You should be selective in your IT applications and work closely with your faculty. Every specialty does not need to try every IT menu choice! Continue to return to the notion that the educational need should drive the technology choice. There may be times you have to say "no" for a variety of reasons. Perhaps the cost of the technology itself is outside your budget that year, but you can always plan to write a grant or make certain to include it in the budget the following year. Your staff may already have too many new projects for the year, so plan to try a pilot before offering to the entire faculty. We have some faculty technology champions who have been essential in helping us to streamline the process of implementation.

Support for faculty goes beyond how many staff members are available. Faculty have to change and diversify while they assume the role of facilitator and must develop the goals of learning, conditions of learning, and methods of instruction.[13] Faculty workloads need to be considered during this development time. It is important when adopting online learning to provide a facilitative environment that promotes human interaction, peer support, and guides socialization. Faculty best-practice models provide an excellent example to peers as to how best to integrate technology into teaching-learning activities. The eLearning Guild surveyed its members in the spring of 2008 for their favorite tips related to strategies for effectively creating, managing, and using synchronous e-learning. The result was 144 tips on synchronous e-learning strategy and research, categorized for blending learning, and for designers, managers, synchronous speakers, and technical production, planning, and preparation.[14] This is a free digital eBook and can be downloaded from the eLearning Guild Web site.

Students, too, must feel supported. Their role transforms from one of passive recipient to one of active learner, a self-motivator who is committed to learning and who possesses self-discipline, and a self-directed learner with time-management skills. Their technology needs to work effectively and efficiently, and they must feel confident in their ability to use these tools independently. Orientation becomes a critical period, and our students are often stressed to make certain that they know how to operate their technology before heading home and feeling isolated.

Table 1 lists possible academic uses of technology with examples and potential staff support suggestions. These technology uses have been categorized as to classroom/lab, learning, research, communication, Web, administrative, and infrastructure. The list is comprehensive, but not exhaustive, and is in no order of priority. The list is not meant to be prescriptive, but rather to offer as a menu approach to those who are planning for IT resources in an educational setting. Some of the applications can be purchased "off-the-shelf" but others require direct programming support, which of course needs to be factored into the decision of whether to purchase or build your own.

Two of the examples mentioned bear further discussion. Knowledge Map is a curriculum management system that has been developed by the Vanderbilt University School of Medicine by two medical students who took a year off from medical school to work with Dr. Anderson Spichard III to develop this advanced curriculum-searching tool that would make their medical education more meaningful.[15] Efforts are currently in progress to interface this tool with the campus-based Blackboard system to integrate the course-based management aspects. In another entrepreneurial venture, Dr. Judith Warren and Dr. Helen Connors from the University of Kansas spearheaded a unique vendor relationship with Dr. Charlotte Weaver from Cerner to develop a "practice" system for nursing students to be able to document into an electronic health record. This unique curricular change was called "SEEDS," which stands for Simulated E-hEalth Delivery System.[16]

After choosing the types of technology, you must then determine your personnel support needs. Support needs will vary depending on the makeup of the personnel you already have on board, ie, each type of IT use does not necessarily require a complete Full-Time Equivalent (FTE) to successfully provide support. A number of factors need to be considered, for example, how many actual classrooms are in your facility that require direct technology support? While one person may be able to support about eight classrooms, this will not be enough if you have scheduled video-streaming to take place in multiple classrooms. During those times, we have resorted to hiring outside camera personnel to provide the necessary camera work and encoding. Your staffing choices may depend heavily on how much is available to you through central administration. Keep in mind that if it is available centrally, then it is available to all faculty members on your campus. There may actually be a financial charge for the service, so find out if there is and how the charge is configured. Will the service be available to you when you need it? Many nursing programs are relying on teaching sessions during evening and weekend hours only to discover that sometimes those support services available centrally are only there 5 days a week from 8 to 5.

Many campuses already have a fairly complex IT Help Desk, but your school needs may not always be met within that environment. Develop a triage system, so that your faculty, staff, and students know who to call locally when specific help is needed, such as configuring a PDA to connect to the campus wireless network.

Table 1
Academic technology uses, examples, and support suggestions

Technology Uses	Examples	Support Suggestions[a]
Classroom/Lab		
"Real" classroom	Computers, Projectors, Microphones, Lighting Controls, SmartBoard technology, Cameras and Infrastructure for Streaming, Polling devices	5, 9
Virtual classroom	Blackboard, Voice-Over Powerpoint, Centra, Videostreaming, MediaSite, Webcasting, Podcasting, MP3 Audio Files of Classes	1, 3, 4, 5, 6, 7, 9
Student computer lab	Lab for application use, testing, teaching for groups	2, 3, 9
Live simulated patient lab	Standardized patients	2, 8, 9
Mannekin simulation lab	Simman, Simbaby, Simchild, task trainers	2, 8, 9
Electronic health record practice systems	SEEDS project	1, 8
Learning		
Multimedia delivery	Computers with high-end video cards, stereo sound cards, and headsets for privacy. Gaming computers work well.	5, 9
Multimedia development	Digital video recording/digitizing equipment. Project management software. Authoring/development tools. Graphics programs. Audio editing programs.	1, 4, 5, 6
Interactive learning development	DxR clinical simulations	1, 6, 4
Virtual reality	Second Life, Augmented Reality	1, 8, 6, 4
Clinical logs	Typhoon, eLog, homegrown systems	1, 9
E-porfolios	Folio	1
Continuing education (CE)	Various CE online programs	3
Web conferencing	WebEx, Centra, Connect, Elluminate, Skype, PolycomPVX	1, 5
Screen capture utilities	Camtasia, Captivate, Lectora Pro, Firefly	1
Research		
Digital library	Authenticated Web access of journals (see campus librarian)	3
Reference materials	PDA, Smartphones, Web access	1
Survey administration	SurveyMonkey, Zoomerang	1, 4

(continued on next page)

Table 1 *(continued)*		
Technology Uses	**Examples**	**Support Suggestions**[a]
Research poster production	Graphics program (Photoshop and/or Illustrator, Paintshop Pro). Poster printer	6
Grant templates	Developed and Connected to Appropriate Databases	4
Proposal reviews	NIH eCommons	1
Communication		
Communication applications	E-mail, Web, Blogs, WIKIS, texting, discussion boards, instant messaging, podcasting, Skype, Journal Clubs, Newsletters, Direction Kiosk, Web 2.0 apps	1, 2, 3, 4, 5, 6, 7, 9
Alumni and development support	Homegrown applications—work with development officer	7, 4
Social networking	Facebook, My Space, Friendster	7
Public relations	You Tube, Public Monitors with Announcements including Weather Status	6, 2, 7
Emergency alert notification	Cell Phone Distribution System (text and audio messages)	4
Web		
Web design, development, evaluation, and updating	Portals with SharePoint Use	7, 6, 3
Web application development	Dreamweaver, Lectora, Flash	7, 6, 3
Sigma Theta Tau virtual chapter support	See University of Phoenix Sigma Chapter	7, 2
Administrative		
Course management systems (CMS)	Blackboard	3, 1
Learning management systems (LMS)	MC Strategies (health systems specific), Saba (generic)	3
Curriculum management	Knowledge Map	4, 3
Online test administration	HESI Testing, NLN Testing, Course-based Testing	2, 3
Test construction, scoring, and analysis	Generally within CMS or LMS	3, 4
Course and faculty evaluations	Either homegrown or within CMS or LMS	3
Online test administration	HESI Testing, NLN Testing, Course based Testing	2
Administrative systems	Financial Aid, Registrar, Billing	4
Faculty/student databases	Working Databases capable of pulling data for Web information	4
Online student applications	Homegrown tied to registrar	4
Student academic advisement	Degree Progress Audit	4

(continued on next page)

Table 1
(continued)

Technology Uses	Examples	Support Suggestions[a]
Clinical placements	Database of where students placed	4
Clinical evaluations	Online evaluation tool that both preceptors and faculty can use	4
Calendar	Open to school, interfaces with university calendar function	4
Room Scheduling	Viewing open, but rights set to schedule by designated individuals	3, 2
Elections	Database results secure by administrator so that voting is anonymous	4
Faculty/staff/student orientation training profiles	Competency-based training	3
Infrastructure		
Hardware/software updates	Hardware on 3-year rotation cycle; Software annual license	9, 3, 1
Data/network security	HIPAA, FERPA guidelines followed, SSL server certificates for all student/ patient data	9, 3, 2
Videoconferencing	Can be point-to-point or many to one designed videoconferencing facility	5, 9

Abbreviations: FERPA, Family Educational Rights and Privacy Act; HESI, Health Education Systems Incorporated; HIPAA, the Health Insurance Portability and Accountability Act; NIH, National Institutes of Health; NLN, National League for Nursing; SEEDS, Simulated E-hEalth Delivery System; SSL, Secure Sockets Layer.
[a] Using nine roles as described in support section.

You may be wondering what constitutes an effective IT support team. There are no magic formulas, but based on my 30 years of technology in higher education, here is the makeup of my team at Vanderbilt:

1. Four nursing informatics faculty members (teach informatics content at the MSN, DNP, and PhD curricular levels and provide peer support)
2. Three administrative support staff (includes computer lab and skills lab support)
3. One director of learning resources (who also programs, supervises the classroom/ lab support areas)
4. Two programmers (including database programming)
5. Two classroom support staff, including video and audio work
6. Two graphic designers
7. One Web developer
8. One skills/simulation director
9. Three network/server/hardware support staff

Together we work as a team, having two overall goals of IT excellence in maintenance and in innovation. We identify annually a technology application that will help to enhance our informatics agenda for the school.

OVERVIEW OF CURRENT ISSUE

Preparing our faculty and students to appropriately use technology in their teaching learning activities is a critical precursor to its actual use. The article by Dr. Carole

Gassert describes technology and informatics competencies across four levels of nurses: beginning nurses, experienced nurses, informatics specialists, and informatics innovators. These competencies must be considered in planning educational programs for health care information technology to be able to transform nursing and health care. In a similar fashion, Dr. Christine Curran describes in depth a faculty development program that resulted in the successful integration of competencies across different levels of a baccalaureate program. At the same time, faculty members were able to upgrade their own technology and informatics skills.

Dr. Patricia Trangenstein describes a comprehensive electronic toolkit for faculty use that can be customized according to the resources of the university. Dr. Karen Ward takes this a step further and describes strategies for success with online learning, using a variety of the tools noted in the electronic toolkit. Dr. Judith Effkin describes the pioneering efforts of the University of Arizona as they converted their doctoral program to a distance-learning format. Lessons learned from all three authors provide a rich environment for others to consider in their integration of technology into nursing education.

Transcultural nursing education is featured in two of the articles. Dr. Jamie Adam describes how an online format can benefit the delivery of transcultural nursing courses that promote culturally competent care. Drs. Sandra Mixer, Marilyn McFarland, and Leigh Ann McInnis promote the use of visual literacy in online environments, and provide the example of a transcultural nursing course that took advantage of the benefits of visual literacy to enhance that course content.

Three of the articles describe applications that are more advanced in nature. The use of PDAs has become more and more complex with the advancing types of hardware, software, and connectivity that have become available. Drs. Renee McLeod and Mary Mays describe these recent innovations and how best to use them for nursing education. Professor Maria Overstreet provides an overview of the use of simulations in nursing education, which as a teaching-learning intervention in nursing curricula has increased greatly during the past decade.[17] Simulations have recently become more important to nursing education because of the increased need for clinical sites, the nursing educator shortage, and concerns about patient safety. The last advanced application described in this issue is survey building. Dr. Jeffry Gordon describes the capabilities provided by recent technology in the development and delivery of surveys, a use that has been further extended with the Web and an interface that back-ends into a server-side database.

SUMMARY

It is an exciting time to be providing quality education to nursing students given the plethora of choice that technology provides. The challenge comes with deciding just what educational outcome you hope to achieve, and designing the appropriate educational milieu to make that happen. Technology should not be used for the sake of playing with technology, but to enhance the learning experience in ways that could not be the same without it. This merging of technology with quality learning requires a myriad of support features, but can be accomplished with thoughtful consideration and planning.

REFERENCES

1. Moody RC, Horton-Deutsch S, Pesut DJ. Appreciative inquiry for leading in complex systems: supporting the transformation of academic nursing culture. J Nurs Educ 2007;46(7):319–24.

2. Alison DA, Deblois PB. The 2008 educause current issues committee. Top-ten IT issues. Educause Review 2008;43(3):36–61. Available at: http://connect.educause.edu/Library/EDUCAUSE+Review/TopTenITIssues2008/46605. Accessed June 1, 2008.
3. Skiba DJ. Nursing education 2.0: twitter and tweets. Nurs Educ Perspect 2008; 29(2):110–2.
4. Wikipedia. Twitter. Available at: http://en.wikipedia.org/wiki/Twitter. Accessed June 1, 2008.
5. Maag M. The potential use of "blogs" in nursing education. Comput Inform Nurs 2005;23(1):16–24.
6. Russell CK, Burchum JR, Likes WM, et al. WebQuests: creating engaging, student-centered, constructivist learning activities. Comput Inform Nurs 2008; 26(2):78–87.
7. Lahaie U. WebQuests: a new instructional strategy for nursing education. Comput Inform Nurs 2007;25(3):148–56.
8. Van't Hooft M. Mobile, wireless, connected: information clouds and learning. Emerging Technologies for Learning 2008;3:30–46. Available at: http://partners.becta.org.uk/index.php?section=rh&;rid=13768. Accessed May 1, 2008.
9. Prensky M. How to teach with technology: keeping both teachers and students comfortable in an era of exponential change. Emerging Technologies for Learning 2007;2:40–6. Available at: http://partners.becta.org.uk/index.php?section=rh&;&catcode=&rid=13904. Accessed May 1, 2008.
10. Skiba DJ. The year in review and trends to watch in 2008. Nurs Educ Perspect 2008;29(1):46–7.
11. Simpson RK. The virtual reality revolution: technology changes nursing education. Nurs Manage 2002;33(9):14–5.
12. Delgado C. Technology in nursing education: five axioms. Nurse Educ 2004; 29(1):13–4.
13. Mancuso-Murphy J. Distance education in nursing: an integrated review of online nursing students' experiences with technology-delivered instruction. J Nurs Educ 2007;46(6):252–60.
14. Elearningguild. 144 tips on synchronous e-learning strategy and research. Available at: www.elearningguild.com. Accessed June 1, 2008.
15. Denny JC, Smithers JD, Armstrong B, et al. Where do we teach what?: finding broad concepts in the medical school curriculum. J Gen Intern Med 2005;20: 943–6.
16. Connors H, Warren J, Weaver C. HIT plants SEEDS in healthcare education. Nurs Adm Q 2007;31(2):129–33.
17. Jeffries P. Getting in S.T.E.P. with simulations: simulations take educator preparation. Nurs Educ Perspect 2008;29(2):70–3.

Technology and Informatics Competencies

Carole A. Gassert, RN, PhD, FACMI, FAAN

KEYWORDS

• Informatics competencies • Health care information technologies

Just a few years ago the health science literature indicated that computers would soon become ubiquitous or be used everywhere to assist in delivering health care. The 2004 call by President Bush for widespread adoption of interconnected electronic health care records[1] has supported increased computer presence in health care. Although more information systems with a computer interface are being implemented, other health care technology applications have also emerged.

Nurse executives have expanded the concept of ubiquitous computing to a broader discussion of using technology for clinical transformation, particularly in acute care settings. By definition clinical transformation is clinical and nonclinical process improvement that is supported by technology. It is important that the technology be seen as supporting these processes and not driving them.[2] Smith[2] identifies categories of technologies needed for clinical transformation as follows:

• information systems—including clinical information systems,
• biomedical monitoring systems—including noninvasive blood pressure and home monitoring devices,
• connectivity or communications—through dial-in or satellite connections,
• patient safety—involving computerized provider order entry, smart intravenous (IV) pumps, barcode medication administration systems, and e-prescribing,
• business and clinical decision support systems,
• education and reference—through patient bedside Internet access, networked patient education systems, and unit-based Internet access for nursing personnel.

As care providers we can expect to see multiple health care information technologies used to achieve clinical transformation. When achieved, clinical transformation should eliminate, for example, situations in which nurses' information is collected for an information system while these same nurses must continue to share additional needed information through shift report or other communications.[3] Further, if

University of Utah, College of Nursing, 10 South 2000 East, Salt Lake City, Utah 84112, USA
E-mail address: carole.gassert@nurs.utah.edu

Nurs Clin N Am 43 (2008) 507–521
doi:10.1016/j.cnur.2008.06.005
0029-6465/08/$ – see front matter © 2008 Elsevier Inc. All rights reserved.

nursing.theclinics.com

information systems are designed to help achieve clinical transformation nurses will not feel these systems impair critical thinking or decrease the quality of care.[4]

HEALTH CARE INFORMATION TECHNOLOGIES

When the phrase health care information technologies is written or verbalized, most health care providers immediately think of information systems. In addition they picture a traditional computer and keyboard located in the "nurses' station" or "physicians' workroom." With the miniaturization of computer chips, numerous technologies have emerged that can support patient care and help the health care industry reach a state of clinical transformation. All of these technologies help to gather or analyze information and will be called health care information technologies (HIT) by this author.

It is not the intent to provide a complete list of health care information technologies. By their nature, HITs are constantly being developed and refined for more efficient collection or analysis of data. Examples of health care information technologies will be presented to show the potential impact of HIT in reaching clinical transformation.

Three examples of health care information technologies, not information systems, used in acute care settings are presented. Bahlman and Johnson[5] describe operating room technologies their institution used to improve communication and workflow in that area. The system combines infrared tracking, a nurse-call system, wireless telephones, and an electronic grease board, which can be viewed on a computer screen or through large monitor screens placed strategically throughout the surgical suite. The system has reduced telephone calls previously made to determine routine information and ensured rapid location of needed equipment, thus streamlining processes.

In a second example, bar-coding technology was implemented to enhance medication administration in a children's hospital in Chicago.[6] Such technology assists nurses in ensuring the five rights in medication administration. The result is improved patient safety through enhanced workflow during medication administration.

Recently Chang and colleagues[7] developed a voice recognition system they tested in the triage area of an emergency department in Taiwan. Nurses were willing to use the system and 99% accuracy in voice recognition was reported. Hopefully this is the beginning of more voice recognition technologies, a relatively untapped means of supporting clinical transformation for nursing with HIT.

Emerging health care information technologies are not just appearing in acute care settings. A few examples of HIT used in nonacute settings will be given. Cheek and colleagues[8] discuss the role that smart technology will play in older Americans aging-in-place, ie, by allowing them to live where they have been with the help of electronic products and conveniences. Smart technology in the home can provide information and communication about the resident's medical condition through a local network connected to a monitoring center. Lighting sensors, motion sensors, environmental controls, emergency assistance, and alerts are examples of smart home technology.

Edge and colleagues[9] discuss an example of how this technology could help an elderly person at high risk of falling get safely to the bathroom during the night. A series of lighting changes would occur automatically during the preset overnight hours if motion is detected and if the person does not return to bed in a specified period of time an alarm would be activated. Smart homes can provide a constantly monitored environment, automate tasks an elderly individual cannot do such as turning on lights or opening curtains, alert care providers of difficulties, and provide prompts to elderly residents to help with compliance to medical routines. It will be interesting to watch how communities designed for the elderly adopt the smart technologies that have to date only been available in more expensive housing as a marketing tactic.

Chang[10] illustrates the use of pocket computers or personal digital assistants (PDA) by adolescents to control and manage their severe asthma. Since PDA-type technology is familiar to most adolescents, they embrace the opportunity to communicate with health care providers about their treatment, to improve their symptoms and to feel in control of their disease.

Health care information technologies can bring acute care and patient home environments or outpatient and home environments together through virtual or telehealth events. To deliver care through telehealth, computerized video equipment is located in patients' homes as well as in either an inpatient or outpatient health care setting. Health care providers can make assessments and recommend follow-up care through interactive video sessions. Courtney and colleagues[11] discuss telehomecare projects that could help to solve issues of health care access and cost related to underserved populations in both rural and urban areas. They further explain that telehomecare events redesign workflows and actually change the point of care for nursing services. Certainly telehomecare events can bring us toward clinical transformation.

Geographic information systems (GIS) represent a health care information technology tool with potential to provide critical information about patients' environmental exposure. Choi and colleagues[12] conducted a study to determine the usefulness of mapping individual's data to environmental data through GIS. They concluded that GIS maps were helpful in describing risk factors and potential health effects.

Nurse's Preparation to use Health Care Information Technologies

All these technologies are great and nurses are prepared to use them! Aren't they? It's hard to believe that in an increasingly technology-rich environment practicing nurses and graduating student nurses are often unprepared to use technology that may be available to them. McBride[13] indicates that the majority of nurses are deficient in needed information technology skills.

The National Agenda for Nursing Education and Practice was published in 1997 to advise the Secretary of the Department of Health and Human Services about nursing informatics needs in education and practice.[14] Five recommendations were made: educate nursing students and practicing nurses in core informatics content; prepare nurses with specialized skills in informatics; enhance nursing practice and education through informatics projects; prepare faculty in informatics; and increase collaborative efforts in nursing informatics.

At the time of the National Advisory Council on Nurse Education and Practice report, most informatics nurses had prepared for their careers in informatics through job experiences, continuing education and self-study.[15] Interestingly, in a 2007 survey of 776 nursing informaticists, 25% of them had received only job training for their informatics roles and 41% indicated they had no formal training in informatics. At the same time, 33% of these nursing informaticists are master's prepared in nursing and an additional 21% have non-nursing master's degrees. Just 17% have a masters' degree in informatics and 2% have a PhD in informatics. Another 12% reported they hold an informatics certificate and an additional 12% of the nurse informaticists are enrolled in either a degree or certificate program in informatics.[16] Noticeably more nurses have been formally prepared in informatics over the past 10 years, but nursing informaticists continue to have a need for formal preparation in their chosen field of practice. The results from the Health Information Management Systems Society survey may reflect the fact that there are only about 12 nursing schools that offer master's-level informatics programs for nurses. That number may decrease as nursing programs switch to offering practice doctorate programs rather than master's programs.

What about practicing nurses? Are they ready to use available and emerging health care information technologies? Few studies are published about practicing nurses' preparation to use HIT. Tannery and colleagues[17] did study practicing nurses' use of information resources once they were exposed to the resources and trained to use them by library personnel. The researchers indicate that if practicing nurses have ready access to knowledge-based electronic information they will use it, a finding important in preparing nurses to function effectively in our evidence-based practice environments.

Obviously, nurses who are exposed to informatics and expected to attain informatics competencies as students would be better prepared to use HIT when they begin their nursing careers. There is recent evidence that informatics skills are being taught in some educational programs but not all.[18] In this study, 266 baccalaureate and higher education programs were surveyed to determine what specific informatics knowledge and skills are currently being taught in baccalaureate and master's-level programs, if faculty are prepared to teach this knowledge, and what the respondents perceive are informatics tools used by practicing nurses.

Astoundingly, half of the baccalaureate programs reported that no informatics subject matter related to 25 specific informatics content areas was included in their curricula. Between a third and a half of baccalaureate programs reported teaching content areas in accessing electronic resources, computer-based patient records, ethical use of information systems, informatics nurse competencies, informatics definitions, hardware and software, evidence-based practice, and information systems in nursing practice, education, management, and research.[18] It isn't clear if students had opportunity or expectations for hands-on experience related to the health care information technologies. This survey suggests that unless they acquire informatics skills independently or have them upon entering their programs, half of the students going into nursing practice upon graduation are not prepared to use critical information systems and technologies needed to bring about a clinical transformation in nursing.

Participants' reports of informatics content areas being taught in graduate nursing programs[18] also raise concern. Only 33% to 38% of graduate programs include accessing electronic records, ethical use of information systems, evidence-based practice, information systems in nursing practice, education management, and research and informatics competences in the curriculum. Less than a third of the graduate programs reporting in the survey include the remaining specific informatics content area. One may argue that we don't need to teach information technology skills to graduate students; they already have needed skills. There is no extensive data on the HIT skills of entering graduate students. But data from McDowell and Xiping[19] indicate that baccalaureate students are not able to increase all needed informatics skills during educational experiences. In their study, students self-reported informatics competencies for 8 years using the Gassert/McDowell[20] Computer Literacy Survey upon entering and exiting their baccalaureate program. Over the years students reported higher levels of skills for word processing, electronic mail, and the World Wide Web both at admission and graduation. Students perceived significantly increased skills in presentation graphics and searching bibliographic databases at graduation. However, they reported continued low-level skills in database searching, spreadsheets, and statistical packages at graduation from their baccalaureate program. Therefore, it is unlikely that entering graduate students have all the health care information technology skills they need for today's practice environments.

A survey of 752 American Organization of Nurse Executives (AONE) members revealed a modest list of critical IT skills needed by nurses at the time of entry into the workforce.[21] Critical IT skills are using e-mail effectively, operating basic Windows applications, searching databases, and knowing nursing-specific software such as bedside charting and computer-activated medication dispensers. Many of our graduates will not be prepared to meet these requirements. Shame on us as educators!

Why are nursing informatics competencies not included in undergraduate and graduate nursing programs? One answer is that faculty do not feel prepared to teach these skills.[18,22–24] McNeil and colleagues[18] found that 57% of responding programs rated their faculty at the novice or advanced beginner level of informatics skills.

A second answer is that nursing accreditation organizations do not list specific outcome criteria for health care information technology[22] for educators or students. For example, the National League for Nursing (NLN) Core Competencies of Nurse Educators published in 2005 have one brief statement about information technologies. It states, "to facilitate learning the nurse educator uses information technologies skillfully to support the teaching-learning process." It will be interesting to see the NLN national standards for nursing students' information technology competence due to be published in 2008.[22]

FORCES DRIVING PREPARATION OF STUDENT NURSES AND PRACTICING CLINICIANS IN INFORMATICS

Alarm about the lack of preparation of student nurses and practicing clinicians to use health care information technology galvanized a small group of individuals to convene a working group of nurses and nurse leaders from industry, education, and government in January 2005 to address the need for nurse preparation in HIT. Hosted by Johns Hopkins University School of Nursing, members of the 1-day session named the project TIGER—Technology Informatics Guiding Educational Reform—and described the platform as follows:

- Ability to use informatics is a core competency for health care providers in the twenty-first century
- Majority of more that 2.8 million licensed nurses lack skills to use online evidence to support evidence-based practice
- Nurse executive leaders lack IT competency and knowledge to lead electronic health record programs at their work
- Nursing education has not included informatics competencies that have been identified as needed in the curriculum
- Numbers of PhD-prepared nurse informaticists are inadequate to prepare the 6000 additional nurse informaticists needed by 2010
- Nursing faculty shortage is compounded by nurses' lack of IT skills to needed to teach required informatics competencies.[25]

The TIGER vision is to (1) allow informatics tools, principles, theories, and practices to be used by nurses to make health care safer, effective, efficient, patient-centered, timely, and equitable; and (2) interweave enabling technologies transparently into nursing practice and education, making information technology the stethoscope for the twenty-first century.[26] To achieve this goal, a 2-day invitational summit was held October 31 and November 1, 2006, in Bethesda, Maryland. More than 100 nursing leaders from over 70 organizations, representing industry, government, nursing, and nursing informatics, developed a TIGER 10-year vision and 3-year action plan. A summary report of the summit is available at https://www.tigersummit.com/Home_Page.html.

Since the summit, nine collaborative teams have been working to accomplish the TIGER vision. Involving more than 260 participants, the teams have met, primarily through virtual meetings, to identify specific goals and assign tasks to members. Focused areas of the nine teams are as follows:

- Standards and interoperability
- Health IT national agenda/HIT policy
- Informatics competencies
- Education and faculty development
- Staff development/continuing education
- Usability/clinical application design
- Virtual demonstration center
- Leadership development
- Patient-focus/personal health record

Collaborative teams expect to finish their work by Fall 2008 and results will be widely disseminated. The Alliance for Nursing Informatics has been the enabling organization for the TIGER initiative since 2007.[27]

Finally, three nursing education programs have listed specific informatics skills as outcome requirements. To meet the outcomes, curricula will be forced to include informatics knowledge and skill. The first program is the clinical nurse leader (CNL), a master's program that prepares individuals to lead in the health care delivery system across all settings.[28] "The CNL assumes accountability for client care outcome through the assimilation and application of research-based information to design, implement, and evaluate client plans of care"[28] (page 3). Information and health care technologies is one of seven areas of core knowledge for the CNL. Under this emphasis area, graduates of CNL programs are expected to

- Use information and communication technologies to document and evaluate client care, advance client education, and enhance the accessibility of care;
- Use appropriate technologies in the process of assessing and monitoring clients;
- Work in interdisciplinary teams make ethical decisions regarding the application of technologies and the acquisition of data;
- Adapt the use of technologies to individual client needs;
- Teach clients how to use health care technologies;
- Protect the safety and privacy of clients relative to use of HIT;
- Use information technologies to increase their own knowledge base;
- Access and critique information sources; and
- Disseminate health care information appropriately using various technologies[28] (page 15)

A second nursing program to stress informatics knowledge and skill is the doctorate of nursing practice (DNP) program. Seven core essentials are listed for the DNP and one of them is "information systems/technology and patient care technology for the improvement and transformation of health care"[29] (page 14). Behavioral outcomes for the DNP relative to health care information technologies are as follows:

- Use HIT in the design, selection, use, and evaluation of programs to evaluate outcomes of care, care systems, and quality improvement;
- Analyze and communicate critical elements necessary to the selection, use, and evaluation of HIT
- Demonstrate ability to develop and execute an evaluation plan involving data extraction from HIT;

- Provide leadership in evaluating ethical and legal issues relative to HIT;
- Select, implement, and evaluate the use of patient care technology; and
- Evaluate consumer health information sources.[29]

The third nursing program to list specific requirements for HIT knowledge and skills is the baccalaureate program. In the document revising the baccalaureate essentials, information management and patient care technology is a content area.[30] Students are expected to be prepared to

- Use information technology and patient data for ethical, effective clinical decision making in providing compassionate patient care;
- Use technologies to assist in effective communication in a variety of health care settings;
- Employ a range of technologies that facilitate patient care, including patient education and patient safety;
- Protect the privacy of patients in relation to the use of information technology;
- Apply safeguards embedded in patient-care technologies and information systems to support a safe practice environment for both patients and health care workers;
- Demonstrate knowledge of regulations that impact the use of technology
- Evaluate patient-care technologies to address the needs of diverse patient populations
- Integrate clinical data from all relevant sources of technology to inform the delivery of care[30] (pages 16–17)

MASTER LIST OF INFORMATICS COMPETENCIES FOR NURSES

In 2002, Staggers and colleagues[31] published the results of a Delphi study to develop a research-based master list of informatics competencies for four levels of nursing practice. Their earlier publication included the preliminary or unvalidated list (305 items) of informatics competencies.[32] The list of validated competencies (281 items) is available at www.nurs.utah.edu/informatics/competencies/htm. The work was done to generate a master list of nursing informatics competencies that could be used to develop core competencies for different nursing specialty groups, a need identified in the NACNEP report to Congress.[14] The work built on efforts initially started by the author while developing and directing the nursing informatics program at the University of Maryland at Baltimore.

Five phases or steps were used to develop and validate the master list of competencies. Initially, competencies were extracted from nursing informatics (NI) literature from 1986-1998, resulting in 1159 items. The author and her colleague Nancy Staggers reviewed the items and inductively placed them into categories and into a database to sort the statements and eliminate redundancies. Three wide-ranging categories emerged. Initially the computer skills category contained 22 subcategories, the informatics knowledge category included 10 subcategories, and the informatics skills category held 25 subcategories of competencies. Subcategories were refined and collapsed as repetitive statements were eliminated. The schema helped to eliminate duplicate statements and identify 313 unique competency statements.

It was alleged by the investigators that not every nurse would be expected to have each of the competencies. Required competencies would be different for novice or for seasoned nurses. Certainly beginning nurses would be expected to have the least comprehensive list of informatics competencies. Nurses who practice in informatics should have many competencies related to systems and data structures that clinically focused nurses would not have. It was also implicit that competencies would be cumulative, ie, more experienced nurses would possess the competencies expected of novice clinicians, informatics specialists would demonstrate competencies accomplished by beginning and more experienced nurses, and nursing informatics innovators would display all of the competencies. Competency statements were placed at the level of practice that described where most nurses would first be expected to demonstrate a particular informatics competency. The levels of nursing practice and the categories and subcategories of competencies form a matrix that describes the progressive nature of the competencies.

At this point in the work process, informatics colleagues from the American Medical Informatics Association Nursing Informatics Work Group were asked to help identify an appropriate level for each of the competency statements. Returned surveys indicated they were unable to complete the task, signifying that a better context for levels of nursing practice was needed. As a third step, the investigators invited four additional colleagues to form an expert panel of six NI specialists to help develop the context needed and place competencies within defined levels of practice. Panel members were as follows: Chris Curran represented nursing practice; Barbara Carty, Ramona Nelson, Rita Snyder-Halpern, and Nancy Staggers were from academia; and Carole Gassert was employed by the government at that time.

Meeting virtually, the panel's work began by refining definitions for the four levels of nurses. With fundamental information management and computer technology skills, the beginning nurse uses existing information systems and other available information to manage their practice. Experienced nurses have proficiency in their domain of interest, eg, cardiac nursing, obstetrics, administration. These nurses are highly skilled in using HIT to support their major area of practice. They see relationships among data elements and make judgments based on trends and patterns within these data. Experienced nurses use current HIT but also work in partnership with informatics specialists to suggest needed improvements for HIT.

The panel defined informatics specialists as registered nurses prepared, at least at the baccalaureate level, with additional knowledge and skills specific to information and HIT. They focus on information needs for nursing practice, including education, administration, research, and clinical practice. Informatics specialists' practice is built on the integration and application of information science, computer science, and nursing science. Informatics specialists use tools of critical thinking, process skills, data management skills (including identifying, acquiring, preserving, retrieving, aggregating, analyzing, and transmitting data), systems development life cycle, and computer skills. Nurses at the highest level of practice are informatics innovators, nurses who are educationally prepared to conduct informatics research and to generate informatics theory. Innovators have a vision of what is possible with HIT, and a sense of timing to make things happen. Innovators lead the advancement of informatics practice and research. They function with an ongoing healthy skepticism of existing data management practices and are creative in developing other solutions. Innovators possess a sophisticated level of understanding and skill in information management and HIT. Innovators understand the interdependence of systems, disciplines, and outcomes, and can finesse situations to maximize outcomes.

Taking the original list of 313 competencies for nurses, the panel added 28 competency statements (3 for the informatics specialist and 25 for the innovator); deleted 41 statements that were duplicates, outdated, or inappropriate; and split four competency statements because they contained more than one behavior. In about 90 statements only the verb was changed to reflect what the panel considered appropriate behavior. Other statements required significant rewording, but about

139 statements remained as abstracted from the literature. There were 304 competency statements for the pilot study.

In the pilot study, the questionnaire was tested with three informatics colleagues: Sue Grobe, Mary McAlindon, and Cheryl Thompson. Respondents took between 45 and 60 minutes to complete the 19-page questionnaire. To validate the competency statements, participants were asked to indicate item importance as an informatics competency (not at all, slightly, required, or critical) and if the statement had been placed at the appropriate level of nursing practice. There were no items added or deleted after the pilot but the wording of seven items was clarified. In addition, one item was split into two statements, yielding a total of 305 items to be validated in the Delphi study.

Using a purposive sample, 110 informatics colleagues recognized as experts, published in the informatics field, prepared at least at the master's level, and having 5 years of informatics practice experience were queried to determine their interest in participating in the study. Questionnaires were mailed to 82 NI experts in Round 1, and 79 met criteria for inclusion in the study. Surprisingly, given the length of the questionnaire, 72 participants (91%) returned questionnaires. They reached consensus on 212 competencies. Seventy participants (97%) validated 49 additional competencies in Round 2. Sixty participants (93%) validated 20 additional competencies in Round 3. To be valid, participants had to reach 80% consensus on item importance and level of competency. In the end, 281 (92%) of the 305 competency statements were accepted as valid informatics competencies, both for their importance and the appropriateness of their level for nursing practice.

In 2007 the list was further validated by Dr. Jieh Chang as part of her doctoral work at the University of Utah (Chang J. Nursing informatics competencies required of nurses in Taiwan: a Delphi method. Unpublished dissertation. University of Utah, 2007). She extended the literature search from 1998 to 2004, abstracted 45 additional items, and added two new subcategories (evidence-based and information literacy) to the informatics knowledge category. Using a Delphi technique to gain consensus, Chang tested a list of 323 informatics competencies with nurse administrators and nurse educators in Taiwan. She asked them to rate each item for importance and level of competency. Participants validated 317 (98%) of her competencies. All but four of the informatics competencies on the Staggers and colleagues'[31] list were validated in Chang's study and most of her added competency statements were validated. The four statements from the work of Staggers and colleagues that were not validated are as follows:

- Explains the use of networks for electronic communication (Level 1)
- Uses application to develop testing materials (Level 2)
- Markets self, system, or application to others (Level 2)
- Serves as a liaison between departments and vendors (Level 3)

Chang's work supports that of Staggers and colleagues[31] and adds competency statements known to be needed for today's practice environments. It would be interesting to validate Chang's updated list with nurses here in the United States.

USING THE MASTER LIST OF INFORMATICS COMPETENCIES FOR NURSES

In the past few years, competency work in informatics has heightened, driven by the desire to use technology for clinical transformation and the concern for patient safety. Judging from the number of citations, much of the reported competency work is based on or uses the list of Staggers and colleagues[31], an excellent use of the master

Table 1
Nursing informatics competencies for beginning nurses, Staggers and colleagues,[31] University of Utah, College of Nursing, Baccalaureate Nursing Program

Category	Functional Subcategory	Competency	Examples of Application
Computer Skills	Administration (Patient Management)	Uses administrative applications for practice management	Searches for patient using UCARE AES Retrieves demographics using UCARE
		Uses applications for structured data entry	Uses pain scales in UCARE Uses Braden scale for pressure ulcers in UCARE Uses patient restraint guidelines in UCARE
Computer Skills	Communication	Uses telecommunications devices (modems, network cards) to communicate with other systems	Completes WebCT assignment Accesses UCARE from remote host Participates in virtual advising for students
		Uses e-mail—creates, sends, responds, uses attachments	Communicates with Student Services Does Apply Yourself online application University of Utah e-mail communication standard—student to administration
		Uses the Internet to locate, download items of interest	Patient resources, disease management My Nursing Lab materials Nursing resources Access UCARE through Internet
Computer Skills	Data access	Uses sources of data that relate to practice and care	Locates "patient data" in UCARE case studies
		Accesses, enters, and retrieves data for patient care	Charts on class activities in UCARE Creates plans of care in UCARE Uses SBAR forms in UCARE Uses fetal monitoring strips in UCARE
		Uses database applications to enter and retrieve information	Enters and retrieves information in UCARE Micromedia database
		Conducts online literature searches	Locates evidence regarding a skill or intervention—some evidence in UCARE

Computer Skills	Documentation	Uses an application to document patient care	Uses UCARE to document results of class activities and simulated patients
		Uses an application to plan care for patients to include discharge planning	Uses UCARE to document plan of care
		Uses an application to enter patient data	Enters vital signs, allergies, admission assessment, and so forth, in UCARE
Computer Skills	Education	Uses information management technologies for patient education	Identifies areas for instruction Conducts education and records outcomes Records teaching plan in UCARE
Computer Skills	Clinical Monitoring	Uses computerized patient monitoring systems	Does critical care clinical in second semester Evaluates fetal monitoring strips in UCARE
Computer Skills	Basic Desktop	Uses multimedia presentations	Leadership course presentation
		Uses word processing	Prepares papers for all classes
		Demonstrates keyboarding skills	Uses keyboard with UCARE
Computer Skills	Systems	Uses networks to navigate systems	Accesses Internet and file servers Uses UCARE to access and chart data Uses WebCt to access and send assignments
		Operates devices peripheral to system	Uses hand-held devices (PDAs), PC tablets for reference materials in clinical settings. Uses bedside terminals in SLC for data capture or exchange in UCARE
		Uses operating systems	Copy, delete, change directories Accesses UCARE through Citrix environment
		Uses existing external peripheral devices	CD-ROMs, flash drives
		Uses computer technology safely	Safely uses UCARE at bedside in Simulation Learning Center (SLC)
		Navigates Windows environment	Manipulate files, determine active printer, access installed applications, create and delete directories
		Identifies appropriate technology to capture required patient data	Fetal monitoring device, physiologic bedside monitor, pulse oximeter, basic EKG, hemodynamic monitoring
		Demonstrates basic technology skills	Creates and prints document (including UCARE) Turn computer on and off, load paper in printer, change toner, remove paper jams

(continued on next page)

Table 1
(continued)

Category	Functional Subcategory	Competency	Examples of Application
Informatics Knowledge	Data	Recognizes the use and importance of nursing data for improving practice	Discusses in first didactic course Receives information in UCARE orientation
Informatics Knowledge	Impact	Recognizes that a computer program has limitations due to its design and capacity of computer	Receives information in UCARE orientation
		Recognizes it takes time, persistent effort, and skill for computers to become an effective tool	Receives information in UCARE orientation
		Recognizes that health computing will become more common	Receives information in UCARE orientation
		Recognizes the computer is only a tool to provide better nursing care and there are human functions that cannot be performed by a computer	Receives information in UCARE orientation
		Recognizes that one does not have to be a computer programmer to make effective use of the computer in nursing	Receives information in UCARE orientation
Informatics Knowledge	Privacy/security	Seeks available resources to help formulate ethical decisions about computing concerns	Uses UCARE
		Describes patients' rights as they pertain to computerized information management	Reviews HIPAA regulations in first semester Applies information by using UCARE
Informatics Knowledge	Systems	Recognizes the value of clinicians' involvement in design, selection, implementation, and evaluation of applications and systems in health care	Discussed in leadership course
		Describes the computerized or manual paper system that is present	Administered student testing with UCARE
		Explains the use of networks for electronic communication	Transfers files with WebCT Accesses UCARE over network
		Identifies basic components of the current information system	Knows components of UCARE

list of competencies. Curran[33] added competencies related to evidence-based practice and abstracted items from the master list to propose a list of nurse practitioner competencies. In 2005, Bickford and colleagues[34] published results from using the competencies to judge outcomes of exposure to the Weekend Immersion in Nursing Informatics continuing education program. Ornes and Gassert[23] used the competency list to evaluate a baccalaureate program to determine if informatics competencies were included in the curriculum.

The Staggers and colleagues'[31] validated list of beginning level informatics competencies is used at the University of Utah to guide the implementation of the Cerner Academic Education Solution clinical information system, named UCARE AES.[35] Of the 37 beginning level informatics competencies for nurses, only 7 are not addressed by using UCARE AES (**Table 1**). From the first day of their nursing education, undergraduate students at Utah are exposed to electronic data management, increasing their preparation for using HIT upon graduation. Because Utah is part of a Cerner AES educational consortium faculty have opportunity to glean new ideas for student learning activities using UCARE. The range of activities is constantly expanding, meeting informatics competency requirements and allowing students to be prepared to use HIT upon graduation.

The TIGER collaborative focused on informatics competencies is pulling together existing competency lists into an overarching framework. The Staggers and colleagues'[31] list is included in that work. The group expects to have its document ready for dissemination by the end of 2008. As nurse educators we need to embrace existing lists of competencies and teach them, not continue to develop more lists that are never implemented. It seems the ball of informatics competencies is in our court and we need to pick it up and run with it, developing educational strategies that will prepare our students to excel as graduates in the health care information technology-rich environments that are developing and will surround us as health care practitioners.

SUMMARY

Use of health care information technology is growing exponentially and nurses need to be prepared to use it. Nursing students continue to graduate without adequate preparation for using HIT. Recent activity to include informatics competencies in program outcomes, as evidenced in the clinical nurse leader, doctorate of nursing practice, and baccalaureate essentials documents will move us toward having our graduates prepared to use HIT. A master list of informatics competencies for nurses has been published and role-specific competencies are appearing in the literature. Nursing educators need to embrace existing competencies and include activities that will prepare our graduates to use health care information technologies that will result in clinical transformation.

REFERENCES

1. Executive Order No. 13335, 69. Federal Register 24059, 2004.
2. Smith C. New technology continues to invade healthcare: what are the strategic implications/outcomes? Nurs Adm Q 2004;28(2):92–8.
3. Ballard E. Exploration of nurses' information environment. Nurse Res 2006;13(4): 50–64.
4. Kossman SP, Scheidenhelm SL. Nurses'perceptions of the impact of electronic health records on work and patient outcomes. Comput Inform Nurs 2008;26(2): 69–77.

5. Bahlman DT, Johnson F. Using technology to improve and support communication and workflow processes. AORN J 2005;82:65–73.
6. Carroll KA, Owen KL, Ward M. Embarking on a journey: implementing bar coding. Comput Inform Nurs 2006;24(5):248–53.
7. Chang P, Sheng Y-H, Sang YY, et al. Developing a wireless speech and touch-based intelligent comprehensive triage support system. Comput Inform Nurs 2008;26(1):31–8.
8. Cheek P, Nikpour L, Nowlin HD. Aging well with smart technology. Nurs Adm Q 2005;29(4):329–38.
9. Edge M, Taylor T, Dewsbury G, et al. The potential for 'smart home' systems in meeting the care needs of older persons and people with disabilities. Available at: www.smartthinking.UKideas.com/SHUPaugust00.pdf. Accessed March 19, 2008.
10. Chang B. Use of personal digital assistants by adolescents with severe asthma: can they enhance patient outcomes? AACN Clin Issues 2003;14(3):379–91.
11. Courtney KL, Demiris G, Alexander GL. Information technology: changing nursing processes at the point-of-care. Nurs Adm Q 2005;29(4):315–22.
12. Choi M, Afzal B, Sattler B. Geographic information systems: a new tool for environmental health assessments. Public Health Nurs 2006;23(5):381–91.
13. McBride AB. Nursing and the informatics revolution. Nurs Outlook 2005;53(4):183–91.
14. National Advisory Council on Nurse Education and Practice. A national informatics agenda for nursing education and practice. Rockville (MD): U.S. Department of Health and Human Services, Health resources and services administration; 1997.
15. Carty B. The protean nature of the nurse informaticists. Nurs Health Care 1994;15(4):174–7.
16. Health Information Management Systems Society. Nursing Informatics Survey. 2007.
17. Tannery NH, Wessel CB, Epstein BA, et al. Hospital nurses' use of knowledge-based information resources. Nurs Outlook 2007;55(1):15–9.
18. McNeil BJ, Elfrink VL, Pierce ST, et al. Nursing informatics knowledge and competencies: a national survey of nursing education programs in the United States. Int J Med Inform 2005;74(11–12):1021–30.
19. McDowell DE, Xiping M. Computer literacy in baccalaureate nursing students during the last 8 years. Comput Inform Nurs 2007;25(1):30–6.
20. Gassert CA, McDowell DE. Evaluating graduate and undergraduate nursing students' computer skills to determine the need to continue teaching computer literacy. Medinfo 1995;8:1370.
21. McCannon' MO, Neal PV. Results of a national survey indicating information technology skills needed by nurses at time of entry into the workforce. J Nurs Educ 2003;42(8):341–9.
22. Fetter MS. Enhancing baccalaureate nursing information technology outcomes: faculty perspectives. [serial online]. Int J Nurs Educ Scholarsh 2008;5(1):1–15.
23. Ornes LL, Gassert C. Computer competencies in a BSN program. J Nurs Educ 2007;46(2):75–8.
24. Nagle LM, Clarke HF. Assessing informatics in Canadian schools of nursing. In: Fieschi M, editor. Medinfo. Amsterdam: IOS Press; 2004. p. 912–5.
25. Weaver CA, Skiba D. TIGER initiative: addressing information technology competencies in curriculum and workforce. Comput Inform Nurs 2006;24(3):175–6.

26. The TIGER initiative. Available at: www.tigersummit.com/about_us.html. Accessed March 23, 2008.
27. DuLong D, Gassert C. Technology informatics guiding education reform: TIGER phase 2: achieving the vision. Comput Inform Nurs 2008;26(1):59–61.
28. American Association of Colleges of Nursing. Working paper on the role of the clinical nurse leader. Available at: www.aacn.nche.edu/Publications/WhitePapers/ClinicalNurseLeader.htm. Accessed August 24, 2004.
29. American Association of Colleges of Nursing. DNP essentials task force report. Available at: www.aacn.nche.edu/DNP/index.htm. Accessed July 12, 2006.
30. American Association of Colleges of Nursing. Revision of the essentials of baccalaureate education for professional nursing practice. Available at: www.aacn.nche.edu. Accessed March 23, 2008.
31. Staggers N, Gassert CA, Curran C. A Delphi study to determine informatics competencies for nurses at four levels of practice. Nurs Res 2002;51(6):383–90.
32. Staggers N, Gassert CA, Curran C. Informatics competencies for nurses at four levels of practice. J Nurs Educ 2001;40(7):303–16.
33. Curran CR. Informatics competencies for nurse practitioners. AACN Clin Issues 2003;14(3):320–30.
34. Bickford CJ, Smith K, Ball MJ, et al. Evaluation of a nursing informatics training program shows significant changes in nurses' perception of their knowledge of information technology. Health Informatics Journal 2005;11(3):225–35.
35. Gassert CA, Sward KA. Phase I implementation of an academic medical record for integrating information management competencies into a nursing curriculum. In: Kuhn KA, Warren JR, Leong TY, editors. MedInfo 2007. Amsterdam: IOS Press; 2007. p. 1392–5.

Faculty Development Initiatives for the Integration of Informatics Competencies and Point-of-Care Technologies in Undergraduate Nursing Education

Christine R. Curran, PhD, RN, CNA[a,b]

KEYWORDS

- Faculty development • Electronic health record
- Nursing education • Technology • Clinical information system
- Informatics competencies

Technology is pervasive. Networked electronic systems have revolutionized our society perhaps even more than the printing press did in its era. The ways in which we communicate, conduct business, learn, travel, and even play are all affected by technology. Academia is no exception. There is an increasing demand for technology-driven techniques and informatics content in curricula; however, faculty members have not

This project was supported by funds from the Division of Nursing (DN), Bureau of Health Professions (BHPr), Health Resources Services Administration (HRSA), Department of Health and Human Services (DHHS) under grant number D11HP03121, Christine R. Curran, PhD, RN, Project Director, and the title "Using Clinical Information Systems at the Point of Care (CIS@POC)" for $904,563. The information or content and conclusions are those of the author and should not be construed as the official position or policy of, nor should any endorsements be inferred by, the DN, BHPr, DHHS or the US government.

[a] UMass Memorial Medical Center, University Campus, H1-753A, 55 Lake Avenue North, Worcester, MA 01655, USA

[b] The Ohio State University College of Nursing, 1585 Neil Avenue, Columbus, OH 43210, USA

E-mail address: curranc@ummhc.org

Nurs Clin N Am 43 (2008) 523–533
doi:10.1016/j.cnur.2008.06.001

kept pace with this educational challenge. Students are outpacing their teachers in the use of networked electronic systems.

A paradigm shift in academia is underway. Faculty can no longer merely be the expert disseminating knowledge; they must shift to a facilitator of learning and create curricula that enable deep understanding of the concepts.[1] Technology can be a facilitator of this needed change. It is an interactive media that requires active learning approaches, but, before it can be used to facilitate learning, one must master the tool itself. Faculty need to develop skills in using electronic applications that can be applied to educational endeavors.

Few universities have formal faculty development programs and even fewer focus on developing skills in the use of technology.[2] Mastering new technology takes time, effort, and resources from the university. Technology involves a hands-on style to education, that is, one in which you learn best by doing.

This article describes one university's attempt to work with faculty to develop their informatics skills to ultimately transform the infrastructure of The Ohio State University (OSU) College of Nursing to include the use of technology in the curricula. Informatics competencies and content, the use of handheld devices, and the use of an electronic health record were introduced into the undergraduate curriculum by working with the faculty teaching six courses. The strategies used to foster development of faculty's skills with technology are discussed.

NEED FOR INFORMATICS AND TECHNOLOGY EDUCATION

The Institute of Medicine[3] named five core competencies needed by all health professionals in 2003. One of these competencies is to use informatics. To give safe and effective care to patients, we must be able to access information at the point of care. Technology not only facilitates this at the individual level but also allows organizations to constantly re-evaluate themselves, streamline processes, raise their quality, and improve business execution. Gates[4] has said that how one gathers, manages, and uses information will determine one's business success. This statement is true for health care as well.

As knowledge workers, nurses need access to patient information and evidence-based content at the point of care. Nevertheless, few schools of nursing have access to electronic health records and other point-of-care technologies to include them into their curricula. Students need to learn the most effective ways to use these tools.

In 2004, the OSU College of Nursing received a Health Resources and Services Administration grant to embed informatics competencies, handheld technology, and an electronic health record into their undergraduate medical/surgical, high acuity, and leadership courses. The goals were to develop an informatics infrastructure, to educate faculty and students in informatics knowledge and skills, and to generate research in informatics. The vision was to create a realistic virtual clinical practice environment for students and to use the technology to transform the way nursing practice was taught and learned.

Several assumptions and beliefs of the author underlie the approaches used in this project:

- One does not learn technology well unless there is a compelling reason to use it.
- Technology is a tool used to improve nursing practice rather than an end in itself.
- Technology needs to be introduced to nurses as students and not when they enter the practice arena.
- Technology can be a vehicle to transform how we teach nursing concepts to students; it requires an interactive engaged learner.

- Creating the most realistic environment for students eases their transition into the actual practice setting.
- Faculty development time needs to be valued and protected for faculty to learn.
- Faculty development activities must to be sensitive to the faculty's historic expert role.
- Experiential learning of technology and informatics concepts by faculty will improve the ability to teach them.
- Informatics competencies are the foundation for learning to effectively use technology to deliver high quality patient care.

Each faculty member involved in the endeavor received a 10% funded effort from the project in an attempt to protect their time for learning and participation on the project.

MODEL FOR FACULTY LEARNING

Fink[5] describes principles of significant learning. For him, significant learning fosters change, is based in real understanding of the concepts and knowledge being conveyed, and provides lasting intelligence on the topic. Six course components are needed to have significant learning: (1) foundational knowledge, (2) application of the new knowledge and skills, (3) integration with existing knowledge, (4) a human dimension, (5) caring, and (6) learning how to learn. Fink recommends the development of learning-centered courses rather than content-focused ones. Thus, the goal of our faculty development efforts was to create an atmosphere focused on learning as opposed to explicit teaching of the informatics competencies and point-of-care technologies being deployed. The faculty would, in turn, teach students using these concepts and tools.

Faculty learning of technology and informatics competencies lends itself well to this framework. The informatics competencies to be integrated into the undergraduate curriculum would provide foundational knowledge for faculty; faculty already possessed the foundational knowledge of nursing. One learns technology best by working with electronic applications, and faculty would be asked to provide assignments for their students to learn each informatics competency required and to test them out (ie, application of new knowledge). Integration with existing knowledge would occur as faculty understood the power of clinical information systems and other point-of-care technologies to enhance information management and delivery of patient care. The human dimension and caring were possible because the core faculty involved were all at the same stage of a novice-to-expert continuum related to informatics content and tools. They were encouraged to collaborate and provide support systems among themselves as well as to solicit support from the project staff and director. We deployed strategies that allowed faculty to learn how to explore software on their own as opposed to a step-by-step instructional process. This approach built confidence in their ability to test out ideas and to be creative using the software. The first opportunity for faculty to learn more about informatics and technology came with the selection of informatics competencies for the graduating Bachelor of Science in Nursing (BSN) student.

INFORMATICS CONTENT AND COMPETENCIES

To embed informatics and technology content into the curricula and to help the faculty's understanding of informatics concepts, our project team solicited faculty participation in selecting informatics competencies for the graduating BSN student. Using the evidence-based work of Staggers and colleagues,[6] the complete list of informatics competencies at all four levels of practice was disseminated to the faculty teaching the six courses targeted by the grant. Additionally, we recruited four practicing nurses, two from an intensive care unit setting and two from a medical/surgical unit, to select competencies they thought the new graduate nurse should possess on entry into practice. This participation was solicited to ensure some level of validation between academia and practice.

After each participant returned his or her individual selections, a matrix was complied that showed each person's choices. Competencies with an 80% agreement among those selecting were accepted for inclusion into the curricula without discussion. For competencies with less than 80% agreement, a meeting was held among all participating faculty and staff nurses. Each item was discussed until a consensus was reached about whether to include it in the revised curricula. Examples of applied competencies were given by the informatics faculty when participants did not understand what was meant by a particular competency. Broad objectives were written to help faculty understand how to translate a given competency for educational purposes. The process improved the faculty's understanding of what each competency meant and how one could design a learning activity to accomplish mastery of a given concept. The ultimate goal was to have each faculty member propose objectives and learning activities that were specific to their course.

Fifty-six competencies were identified as outcomes for the BSN nursing program. The faculty selected all 37 of the level one competencies, 18 of the level two competencies, and 1 level three competency from the original master list developed by Staggers and colleagues.[6] Level two competencies in the original study were agreed upon for the experienced nurse and level three for the nurse informatics specialist; however, as people in our society progress in their informatics proficiency, it is expected that competencies will shift down in the level of sophistication needed to execute them. Thus, it was not surprising that some level two competencies were selected. The level three competency related to virus detection, and the faculty believed that this was an important skill for all system users.

Once the final list was compiled, faculty were asked to analyze the list to see if any competencies should be prerequisites to the program and which competencies were already being taught in the curricula. Faculty selected 18 of the competencies as prerequisites to entry into the undergraduate program. All but one of the identified prerequisites came from the level one competency list of Staggers and colleagues.[6] Faculty gave examples of 11 nursing informatics competencies that were currently being taught in the undergraduate medical/surgical, high acuity, or leadership courses. That left 27 competencies needing to be added to the curriculum.

For each new competency, the faculty discussed which course seemed most appropriate to introduce the informatics competency; courses later in the curriculum could be used to reinforce each concept. All of the six courses added new competencies to their curriculum. Three courses involved students at the sophomore level, one course was a junior year course, and the remaining two courses affected senior students. **Table 1** depicts the new competencies added by student year within the curriculum. Faculty gained a working knowledge about each competency as they were discussed; faculty development was a planned byproduct of revising the curricula.

INTRODUCTION OF POINT-OF-CARE TECHNOLOGIES

Concurrent with the work to determine nursing informatics outcomes for the BSN program, the project provided funds for the purchase of an electronic health record for the

Table 1
New informatics competencies added by year in the BSN program

Competency	Student Level		
	Sophomore	Junior	Senior
Uses administrative applications for practice management	×	—	—
Uses applications for structured data entry	×	—	—
Accesses, enters, and retrieves data used locally for patient care	×	—	—
Uses database applications to enter and retrieve information	×	—	—
Uses an application to document patient care	×	—	—
Uses an application to plan care for patients to include discharge planning	×	—	—
Uses an application to enter patient data (eg, vital signs)	×	—	—
Performs basic trouble-shooting in technology	×	—	—
Acts as an advocate of system users including patients or clients	×	—	—
Applies monitoring system appropriately according to the data needed	×	—	—
Evaluates computer-assisted instructions as a teaching tool	×	—	—
Recognizes the use and/or importance of nursing data for improving practice	—	×	—
Extracts data from clinical data sets	—	×	—
Extracts selected literature resources and integrates them to a personally usable file	—	×	—
Discusses the principles of data integrity, professional ethics, and legal requirements	—	×	—
Describes ways to protect data	—	×	—
Assesses the accuracy of health information on the Internet	—	×	—
Assists patients to use databases to make informed decisions	—	×	—
Supports efforts toward development and use of a unified nursing language	—	×	—
Promotes the integrity of nursing information and access necessary for patient care within an integrated computer-based patient record	—	×	—

(continued on next page)

Table 1 (*continued*)	Student Level		
Competency	Sophomore	Junior	Senior
Provides for efficient data collection	—	×	—
Recognizes the value of clinicians' involvement in the design, selection, implementation, and evaluation of applications, systems in health care	—	—	×
Uses applications to manage aggregated data	—	—	×
Uses data and statistical analyses to evaluate practice and perform quality improvement	—	—	×
Describes general applications available for research	—	—	×
Defines the impact of computerized information management on the role of the nurse	—	—	×
Participates in influencing the attitudes of other nurses toward computer use for nursing	—	—	×

College of Nursing as well as a plan to introduce handheld devices for faculty and students. To pace the learning requirements for faculty and students, the electronic health record was introduced to faculty in year 1 and to students in year 2 of the project; the handheld devices were given to faculty in year 2 and to students in year 3. The goal was to allow time for the faculty to become proficient in the use of the technology before providing these tools to students.

Clinical Information System

Virtual cases were designed to populate the database of the clinical information system/electronic health record.[7] Each of the six courses was analyzed for existing clinical cases and vignettes. A matrix was used to outline all clinical cases across the courses. Faculty were then brought together to agree on a core set of clinical case scenarios that would serve as a standard set of virtual clinical patients within the electronic health record. Cases were outlined on paper and supporting data and documentation entered into the system. Once the cases were fully developed within the clinical information system software, they became the content used to teach faculty how to navigate the electronic health record.

Faculty members were taught the components of an electronic health record through hands-on classes using the software and queries about cases to navigate the system. Sessions were not explicitly labeled faculty development. Faculty was brought together to review the content of the electronic health record to ensure that sufficient data existed for teaching purposes with their students. A byproduct of this "exploration" was that faculty learned to navigate the system to find all of the information they needed to convey in class. This approach reinforces the belief that technology is a tool that can facilitate learning and practice but is not an end in itself. This technique would not work in an actual practice setting because patients' lives depend on timely access to the information contained in an electronic health record.

To further encourage use of the cases in their class, faculty was asked to generate additional clinical data to embellish the cases when they were found to be lacking adequate depth (ie, to add content for the concepts being introduced in their course). It became apparent to the faculty that the amount of data available in an electronic health record far exceeds that typically used in case presentations in education today. The richness of the data in the virtual electronic health record more closely resembles the information available in actual practice. Students have more robust information to make decisions, and faculty can begin to teach more effectively about subtle as well as overt patient findings and their implications.

To encourage faculty to explore how they might use the electronic health record with students, the software was placed on their office machines, and they were given remote access to the system from home. Information systems technical support staff, a systems administrator (who builds the cases and content within the software), and myself as an informatics faculty and project director were available to support faculty as they learned to use the system. Technical support was critical, because learning could not take place if faculty members were frustrated with making the technology work; likewise, informatics support was crucial to help translate concepts into technology and software-ready forms that free faculty to be creative in teaching strategies.

Teaching methodologies and learning activities and exercises needed to be developed for each of the new competencies targeted for all six courses. Some of these competencies were best achieved by using the electronic health record in class or for homework assignments. An expectation was set for the project that each faculty should add one new student activity per quarter that involved use of technology, such as building a patient's care plan in the electronic health record. The activity had to be achieved to address a required informatics competency for the course.

Individual meetings were held with each faculty member responsible for one of the courses in the project. Objectives and content for each course were reviewed. Faculty was coached about possible teaching strategies and assignments that could be used to embed the new informatics content and skills. Because there are multiple ways that each competency can be explicated, mock ups of the assignments or practice sessions using the electronic health record or Internet helped faculty make final selections for new activities and assignments for each course. Faculty began to see how they could demonstrate relationships between concepts using their new skills.

Handheld Devices

Our goal with handheld devices was to give students and faculty access to reference materials at the point of care. The dean of the college generously decided to fund the software for the personal digital assistants (PDAs). She also offered to buy a PDA for any faculty member not on the grant as long as they agreed to use them with students in their courses. Ultimately, this funding helped to create a larger pool of faculty interested in using technology in academia who bonded around a common interest. They began to exchange ideas and classroom exercises among themselves.

To assist with faculty buy-in, project faculty participated in the selection of the software packages. Once agreement was reached on specific software, they were asked to test the potential software for one quarter before the package was purchased for students. For faculty to "pilot test" the software, they needed to learn how to operate the PDA, what each application contained and how to navigate that application, and how these applications could be used in their courses. Formal sessions on the use of PDAs were held. Several interactive sessions with visiting professors occurred, the information technology and project staff assisted, and a doctoral student proficient in PDA use took the proposed software and mapped out sample exercises that could be used for a course at each level (sophomore, junior, and senior). Learning occurred through hands-on discovery, exploring the sample assignments generated by the doctoral student, from the formal interactive classes, and as a byproduct of being on the grant with the expectation to use them in their courses. One of our technical desktop support staff became proficient in the use of the PDAs and provided technical support for the faculty using these devices.

INTEGRATION OF INFORMATICS CONTENT, TECHNOLOGY, AND SKILLS IN COURSES

Competencies and point-of-care technologies were translated into learning content, activities, and outcomes for the students. In the sophomore year, the following content, activities, or both were added to the curriculum by the end of year 3 of the project: an introduction to structured terminologies (given in the form of a computer-based learning module), use of an electronic care plan constructor, an introduction to more sophisticated online literature search strategies (eg, the use of the Cochrane database), an introduction to structuring data for analysis, a formal interactive class and assignments using RefWorks (our reference management software product), and an introduction to handheld technologies and the clinical software available on each device. A suite of clinical reference software products (ie, a medical dictionary, an evidence-based practice reference, a medication reference text, a laboratory and diagnostics text, and a set of clinical calculators) was loaded onto each faculty's and student's device. Exercises and homework assignments were created to use the PDAs in coursework, and students found them invaluable in the clinical settings. Students participated in focused simulation exercises that embedded informatics content and competencies. The electronic health record was used with almost every simulation to model the actual practice environment. Students were expected to look up needed results and clinical data as well as document their assessments and care.

The junior students were introduced to evaluation of Web sites, information on minimum data sets, ways to obtain different information sources on a specific topic within E-portfolios, use of E-mail between clinicians and patients, and more handheld technology applications. Students at this level participated in their first case-based, high-fidelity simulation, and over the course of the quarter each student participated in four simulations. Students received a homework assignment that involved a review of a clinical case in the electronic health record and were requested to look up the best practices for a patient with that diagnosis. This case would be used for the simulation the next day. Once in the laboratory, students received a "bedside" report, had access to the electronic medical record, and were asked to provide care for their "patient" (generally with some problem to be solved during the scenario). Results arrived during the simulations, orders were placed, and documentation was expected as care was delivered. Student could use their PDAs to look up information that they needed to provide care. The simulation experience closely resembled actual practice and demonstrated the use of point-of-care technologies.

Senior students gained knowledge and experience in constructing data displays for analysis (multiple parameters, grid analysis, pattern detection, and correlation of patient information with underlying pathology), aggregating data and turning data into information. An electronic Quality Improvement exercise was constructed using the clinical information system. Content on benchmarking and scorecards was added to the leadership course, and a skills laboratory exercise was developed to help students learn how to prioritize and delegate care as well as to effectively make patient assignments. High-fidelity simulation experiences involved more complex patient scenarios, and, as always, the electronic health record was used as the foundation to get to know the patient.

FORMAL FACULTY DEVELOPMENT INITIATIVES

Recognizing the need for foundational informatics knowledge and skills of the faculty, planned formal faculty development sessions were built into the project budget. The initial goal was to deliver one formal "class" in the fall and one in the spring of each year of the project (six total sessions); however, a decision was made to "front load" the classes to build a stronger knowledge base for faculty. Although the faculty members involved in the project were expected to attend, the sessions were opened to all faculty within the College of Nursing. A basic premise for these sessions was that each must have an interactive and hands-on component to them to engage the faculty in learning.

We were able to deliver eight formal faculty development sessions over the 3-year project period. Topics were targeted at skills needed by all faculty within the college. In year 1, sessions on evaluation of Web sites using the Health on the Net criteria, use of reference management software, the need for structured terminology in clinical information systems (given by Dr. Judith Warren of Kansas University), and the use of high-fidelity simulation (presented by Dr. Pam Jeffries of Indiana University) were conducted. In year 2, we focused on the use of PDAs. Three interactive presentations occurred: (1) an introduction to use of the handheld device, (2) PDA use in the classroom (given by Dr. Linda Goodwin of Duke University), and (3) a lecture entitled "Mobile Technology: On the Brink of Transforming Nursing Education" (presented by Dr. Fran Cornelius of Drexel University). The focus of year 3 was on dissemination of our work. We gave two internal presentations to all faculty on the project—one on the vision, planning, and execution of the project and the other on development of the cases for the electronic health record. Content from each session was used to reinforce some aspect of the project work and helped to build the faculty's confidence in their ability to use technology and informatics content to achieve student learning of nursing principles and practices, especially in areas of information management.

LESSONS LEARNED

Limited evidence-based literature exists in nursing on the topic of faculty development. Matthew-Maich and colleagues[8] found that faculty members experience a sense of evolving as educators through a community of faculty development. Likewise, we found that having a core group of faculty learning new skills together builds a community of learning within the faculty. Support and resources from the dean were also crucial to our success as well as having grant funding to implement our vision.

Williams and colleagues[9] reviewed faculty development initiatives to promote geriatrics teaching. Features that were found effective in fostering sustained change in clinical teaching included selecting a small group of "star" educators to develop, cultivating projects that led to clinical or educational improvements, and creating ongoing working relationships among faculty. The OSU project did all three of those things. A small core group of faculty taught courses targeted by the grant (our stars), projects were created to master their skills and to convey informatics content and competencies to students, and faculty built new relationships with their peers as a result of the need to work together on this project.

Foley and colleagues[10] identified the following conditions as necessary for an effective faculty development plan:

- Teaching is valued within the organization.
- Faculty is a crucial university resource and should be helped to develop and be successful.
- A formalized, structured, goal-oriented program is necessary to support faculty professional growth.
- Faculty development needs to be connected to the institution's reward structure.
- Support from colleagues in becoming excellent teachers is an investment in success.
- Faculty need to have ownership of the development program.
- Administrative support for faculty development is essential.

Although these conditions existed at OSU, the real driver of faculty learning in my opinion was a clear expectation to embed new informatics content and skills into the curricula. The grant helped to explicate the vision, structure the timelines, and provide resources. It took faculty awhile to understand and buy in to the vision. A real turning point for them was when we presented our first set of reports at a North American conference and they saw the positive reaction of the audience to their work. Although the college had rewarded faculty for their efforts, external peer recognition was the most important reward for faculty.

SUMMARY

Boyden[2] has claimed that the paucity of nursing informatics content in the current curricula has resulted in the lack of faculty development programs on this topic. Faculty must grasp the importance of using technology to facilitate learning and knowledge of informatics concepts and skills. Informatics is the science of how one turns data into information and ultimately knowledge.

Technology is not only a tool one needs to learn how to use to maximize knowledge but also one that can be used to transform learning. Only when faculty understand the potential of the electronic health record and other technologies to manage individual and patient population information can they effectively use this tool for educational gains. Faculty development in informatics and technologies is crucial to the successful future of nursing practice.

REFERENCES

1. Magnussen L. Applying the principles of significant learning in the e-learning environment. J Nurs Educ 2008;47(2):82–6.
2. Boyden KM. Development of new faculty in higher education. Journal of Professional Nursing 2000;16(2):104–11.
3. Institute of Medicine. Health professions education: a bridge to quality. Washington, DC: National Academies Press; 2003.
4. Gates W. Business at the speed of thought: a digital nervous system. New York: Warner Books; 1999.
5. Fink LD. Creating significant learning experiences: an integrated approach to designing college courses. San Francisco (CA): Jossey-Bass; 2003.
6. Staggers N, Gassert C, Curran C. A Delphi study to determine informatics competencies for nurses at four levels of practice. Nurs Res 2002;51(6):383–90.

7. Curran CR, Elfrink V, Mays B. Building a virtual community for use in nursing education: the Town of Mirror Lake. J Nurs Educ, in press.
8. Matthew-Maich NM, Mines C, Brown B, et al. Evolving as nurse educators in problem-based learning through a community of faculty development. Journal of Professional Nursing 2007;23(2):75–82.
9. Williams BC, Weber V, Babbott SF, et al. Faculty development for the 21 century: lessons from the Society of General Internal Medicine—Hartford Collaborative Centers for the Care of Older Adults. J Am Geriatr Soc 2007;55(6):941–7.
10. Foley BJ, Redman RW, Horn EV, et al. Determining nursing faculty development needs. Nursing Outlook 2003;51:226–31.

Electronic Toolkit for Nursing Education

Patricia A. Trangenstein, PhD, RN-BC

KEYWORDS

• Nursing education • Distance education
• Educational technology

"Technology Changed Today...Have You Caught Up?"
—(Unknown)

For years, the mainstay of nursing education has been face-to-face encounters. Currently no technology exists that can precisely replicate a face-to-face class, yet the explosion in information and knowledge compels nurse educators to use these encounters more efficiently. "Today, staying in place means falling behind and no one can afford to do that in a technology-driven world".[1]

Since the introduction of the World Wide Web in the early 1990s, there has been an explosion of Web-based educational tools. More and more nursing programs are incorporating Web-based technologies into their curricula. The challenge for nurse educators is to assimilate the knowledge and expertise to understand and appropriately use these electronic educational tools to supplement and enhance student learning.

There are several distinct advantages to electronic educational activities because of the ability to preserve or archive the materials. Electronic course materials can be accessed 24 hours a day, 7 days a week from any Internet connection, and students can review materials as often as is necessary. This article describes various electronic educational tools and their uses. Nurse educators can then select appropriate applications that are supported by their institution to construct their own "toolkit."

IN ADVANCE

Choosing a technological solution before analyzing the educational activity is rarely successful. Instructors should identify the problem, profile the learners, and define the objectives before adopting any electronic educational tool. Chickering and Gamson[2] identify seven effective educational practices that are well suited to Web-based education. They are

• "Encourage contact between students and faculty
• Develop reciprocity and cooperation among students

Vanderbilt University, School of Nursing, 461 21st Avenue South, Nashville, TN 37240-2549, USA
E-mail address: trish.trangenstein@vanderbilt.edu

Nurs Clin N Am 43 (2008) 535–546
doi:10.1016/j.cnur.2008.06.004
0029-6465/08/$ – see front matter © 2008 Elsevier Inc. All rights reserved.

nursing.theclinics.com

- Encourage active learning
- Give prompt feedback
- Emphasize time on task
- Communicate high expectations
- Respect diverse talents and ways of learning."

Matching the appropriate technological solution to the proposed educational activity commonly involves consulting with instructional designers and/or local technical support to decide if implementation is feasible.

COURSE MANAGEMENT SYSTEMS: A VIRTUAL CONTAINER

In the current day and age it is unlikely that only one electronic educational tool will be used in a given course. Common tools are frequently integrated into suites called course management systems (CMS). The Western Cooperative for Educational Telecommunications (WCET) has identified over 15 different course management systems on its EduTool Web site.[3] This site provides feature-by-feature product comparisons and a decision tool for selecting an appropriate product.

Course Management Systems Learner Tools

In general, features contained within a CMS can be categorized as learner tools or course maintenance tools (**Table 1**). The learner tools include collaboration and student productivity components. To facilitate discussion and dialog between instructors and learners and among learners, collaboration tools include both synchronous (real-time interactive chat, whiteboard) and asynchronous (discussion board) methods that are primarily text based. Chats allow for real-time interaction while asynchronous discussions allow participants time for reflection and deliberation. Electronic collaboration tools can be used for information sharing, processing ideas, tutorials, virtual office hours, improving learners' communication skills and file sharing, and group building.[4]

Because contributors do not have to purchase additional software or hardware, Instructional Electronic Chats (IECs) are an economical way of providing prompt feedback, encouraging contact among participants, and developing cooperative learning communities. However, the use of real-time (IECs) presents some unique challenges.[5] Creating a balance between strictly instructor-controlled dialogs and multiple, confusing, simultaneous conversations requires expertise and skill. Nurse educators can adopt protocols or communication conventions to minimize confusion and misunderstanding. Smith[6] refers to this as "chatiquette" and recommends the use of rules such as "?" to indicate a question, "!" to provide a comment, and "///" to indicate a completed comment. Typed responses should be "chunked" or split into short, easily readable elements to improve communication flow and minimize lengthy breaks or disjointed dialog. Participants proficient with chat rooms, often use acronyms or emoticons to express feelings or to accelerate dialog. Lists of Internet acronyms and text emoticons can be found on various Web sites such as Netlingo[7] or Windweaver's Recommended Emoticons for Email Communication.[8]

Other learner tools include student productivity aids such as an assignment section and a course calendar. The learner's ability to bookmark or identify the last place visited in the electronic course is beneficial. And finally, a digital drop box allows the instructor and a given learner to exchange files. After the learner submits the assigned file to the instructor, the instructor can retrieve and review/grade the assignment and return it to the individual student. While electronic files can be submitted as attachments to an email sent to the instructor, the use of a digital drop box avoids the

Table 1
Selected features of a course-management system

LearnerTools			Course Maintenance tools		
Collaboration tools	Productivity aids	Administrative tools	Communication Tools	Course content tools	Student Assessment tools
Chat	Assignments	Authentication	Announcements	Customizable templates	Online grade book
Discussion board	Bookmarks	Course replication	Distribution Lists	File management	Testing
File exchange	Calendar	Registration	E-mail	Multimedia capability	Portfolios
Group work	Digital drop box	Role assignment	—	—	Surveys
Whiteboard	—	Student tracking	—	—	—

locating, sorting and/or filtering of submitted course materials from accumulated emails and prevents the accidental return of one student's electronic files to another student.

Course Management Systems Course Maintenance Tools

Other course management systems tools help to manage the more routine tasks of class management such as communication with learners, access to course files, and online student assessments. In addition, various administrative tools allow the instructor to manage users and student enrollment; copy, import, or archive course materials from one term to the next; assign course roles; and track student access.

Course files located in a CMS are not restricted to text only. The ability to add graphics images and audio and video files can engage the learner and allow instructors to address diverse learning styles. The limiting factor is the bandwidth (Internet connection) available to the learner. Students who use dial-up access need a text-based-only format to ensure that they have access to course materials. Also, the addition of multimedia in course files frequently requires the learner to download and install additional players to view these materials.

The addition of multimedia elements increases file sizes and if mounted to the CMS server can lead to server congestion. A better practice is to copy course files containing multimedia to a separate server and provide links to that site within the CMS. This practice prevents bottlenecks and the slowing or interruptions of services.

A study of over 700 faculty and staff at the University of Wisconsin[9] supports anecdotal evidence that instructors' use of a CMS tends to concentrate on the content presentation tools. Instructors tend to look upon the CMS as an organizational tool for their course and are more comfortable adopting strategies with lower learning curves. However, this study also showed that an indirect result of using a CMS was that, over time, instructors began restructuring their courses and changing the way they taught as they discovered new ways to use the tools in their classes.

LEARNING MANAGEMENT SYSTEMS

A product similar to the CMS is the learning management system (LMS). While these two products are often confused, they really serve significantly different purposes. The CMS is a repository for course material as previously mentioned, whereas the LMS contains course online lessons that can be sequenced for presentation. The LMS can be programmed so that before the user sees topic B, he or she must successfully complete topic A. The LMS can track performance within a specific course, keep records of that performance, and send a completion report to an instructor or employee's supervisor.

Typically, universities use a CMS such as Blackboard to post course content that is normally addressed in face-to-face classes, whereas businesses and corporations (such as a hospital that is responsible for employee on-the-job training) will use an LMS environment. This environment can also track continuing education units and certifications and alert the client and supervisor when certifications are expiring.

A number of companies have created LMS environments. Some of these are fairly generic, such as the SABA Learning Suite or Trivantis' Coursemill. In those, all material must be populated by those in charge of instruction. Other systems embed access to specific content within their system. HealthStream's Learning Center, for example, provides access to articles of interest to the health care profession. If one acquires their system one also acquires access to these articles. This is extremely useful to organizations that do not have the resources to secure access to all of the journals students may find of interest in a course.

LMS systems tend to be a lot more processor and disk drive intensive than their CMS counterpart. Often entire courses and their associated media (digital videos for example) are posted inside the LMS. It is therefore important to scale the size of the server the LMS resides on to the client load that the organization requires. Undersizing the computer, the bandwidth connection, and the disk drives will result in slow-loading courses that will just frustrate the users. Unlike CMS systems that are run on client-controlled servers, LMS systems can also be hosted and space rented. The advantage to renting is that the client site does not need local expertise to administer a server or the bandwidth to deliver the instruction.

ADDITIONAL TOOLS

Table 2 lists the electronic educational tools found in most CMS/LMS as well as additional Web-based applications that can be adopted. As a general rule, the more simultaneous, natural interaction required, the more expensive the solution. Many of these applications require the institution to purchase additional software and the participants to acquire additional hardware such as Web cameras. If audio interaction is desired, participants should purchase headsets (earphones with an attached microphone) to minimize noise and prevent reverberations. More technical support and additional training are usually required. These supplementary tools can be classified into six categories: collaboration, communication, discussions, presentation of materials, content development, and clinical education.

Collaboration Tools

Wikis are a unique collaboration tool where multiple participants become contributing authors. Participants freely manage, edit, and organize content on a Web site using a standard Web browser. Changes are tracked and become part of the site's record. Weblogs (blogs) on the on the other hand, are Web sites maintained by an individual usually on a particular subject. The author provides his or her opinion and allows others to leave their comments. Both of these tools can be used for group work, peer review, and project development. While these may be excellent spontaneous tools for sharing knowledge, if there are little restrictions, constructive dialog can collapse into inflammatory or inaccurate commentaries.

Communication Tools

Instant messaging (IM) and peer-to-peer networks (P2P) are two communication tools worth mentioning. With instant messaging two individuals exchange real-time text messages that allow for quick questions and clarifications. Each participant must register and provide a unique user name. Many instructors use this format for virtual office hours.

Similar to instant messaging, peer-to-peer networks connect two locations over the Internet but allow the addition of two-way audio and video if Web cameras and headsets are provided. Generally, there are no additional software costs for these applications. Products such as Skype (Skype Technologies S. A., Luxembourg) can be used to connect instructors at the home institution with either preceptors or students at a distance for virtual site visits or advising. Because of this direct network connection between two computers, the issue of firewall barriers often encountered with external health care organizations can be circumvented.

Table 2
Electronic educational toolkit

Educational Activity	Solution	Comments
Assessment/Evaluation	Online Testing via CMS/LMS LMS can sequence instruction, create certificates, track certifications	Test score automatically inserted into gradebook
	Online Survey via CMS/LMS	Statistics computed
Clinical Log	—	Web-based system to tracks students' clinical encounters, can capture at point of care with PDA and upload
Collaboration	Assign groups within CMS	—
	Weblogs (blogs)	Spontaneous tool for sharing knowledge, individual provides his or her opinion on a given subject and allows others to leave their comments.
	Wikis	Allows all participants to create and edit a Web site
Communication	E-mail/announcements via CMS/ LMS	One-to-one or one-to-many
	E-mail distribution lists	Primarily text, one-to-many
	Instant Messenger	Primarily text, can add voice and video, one-to-one or can branch into chat
	Peer-to-peer networks (P2P) Voice and video over Internet, eg, Skype (Skype Technologies S.A., Luxembourg)	Point-to-point (no more than 2 at one time) Other features may include instant messaging, file transfer, direct connection circumvents firewall issues, headset and Web cam required
Discussions	Discussion Board	Asynchronous—text only
	Chat	Synchronous—text only
	Phone conferencing	Synchronous—voice only, difficult to record session
	Web Conferencing/Meeting Type I: Connect to Web site, audio over phone	Real-time interaction, may require download of application, hosting charges incurred
	Web conferencing/meeting Type II: includes Voice over Internet Protocol (VOiP)	Real-time interaction using digital audio, headset required, additional site licensing costs usually per seat, may require download of application, desktop application sharing available
Physical Demonstrations	Streaming digital video	Requires tech support, end product should be housed on a multimedia server

(continued on next page)

Table 2 (continued)		
Educational Activity	**Solution**	**Comments**
Presentation of Material	Presentation software. Easy: PowerPoint. Difficult: course content development tools	Learner can view materials as frequently and when they want. The "difficult" approach typically requires development designers with additional expertise
	Voice over Presentation	Instructor's voice is captured, narrating each slide. Voice is synchronized to each slide. Cannot pause when recording, must capture in one take. Cannot capture live face-to-face class. End product should be posted on multimedia server
	Desktop Screen Recorder	Captures mouse strokes on desktop, useful for demonstrating other software programs such as spreadsheets or statistical packages. Can interrupt/pause capture. Cannot capture live face-to-face class. Additional cost for site license.
Submission of Assignments	E-mail attachment Small classes or small (text) files	Time stamped, learners should use a standard subject line when submitting, ie, Course#LastNameAssigmentNameor #
	Digital Drop box Large classes or large file sizes	Time stamped, learner must click submit to post file

Abbreviations: CMS, course management system; LMS, learning management system.

Web Conferencing

While asynchronous material presentation has long been a mainstay of distance learning, there is a growing family of products that allow the instructor and students to meet online synchronously (at the same time), share each other's desktop, and hear each other speak. Classes of this type are of a more traditional nature where an instructor presents material (including PowerPoint [Microsoft Corporation, Redmond, WA] slides) and engages the students in a live verbal discussion. Although WebEx made this technology popular, there are now a variety of products that accomplish similar tasks. Examples of competitive products in this area include SABA Centra, Microsoft LiveMeeting, GoToMyMeeting, Adobe Connect, and Elluminate Live!

All of these products have two components. The first allows the users to share whatever is on their desktop. Typically the faculty member's desktop is shared with PowerPoint slides. As the instructor brings up a new slide, the students then see that new slide on their computers, all at the same time. If the students are presenting projects, these applications allow the faculty member to turn the system over to the presenting students to show their desktop to the class. But these systems are not limited to PowerPoint slides. Web pages and PC-based applications can also be demonstrated. Because of bandwidth limitations, the users should avoid sharing full motion multimedia animations or videos. These tend to look very jerky in these applications. Likewise the users need to be aware of color palette limitations. Shared photos with a million-color color palette may look very pixelated with unusual color mappings.

The second key feature of these products is the ability to share audio. The students cannot only hear the instructor, they can raise their hands online and talk back to the instructor. They can also talk to each other. This voice-over IP (VOIP) feature is an emerging technology. It requires a headset with a microphone. Bandwidth limitations at the server site, client (student or faculty) sites, and general Internet traffic can all interfere with audio quality and throughput. Although this technology is improving every day, if students are having audio issues the instructor may be better off using telephone conference calling for the audio component. While this can be expensive (VOIP, on the other hand, is free to the user) you do frequently get what you pay for. Keep in mind that although only 1 student in 10 may have audio problems, if there are 10 students in the "room" the loss of that 1 student and the time it takes to determine a solution can destroy a class session.

Additional key features of these products allow the students to raise their hands, generate class lists so the instructor knows who is online, and text chat capabilities to augment audio capabilities. A few products allow the user to take a test online, allow the instructor to divide the class into separate distinct sections, permit the students to share video of themselves from their desktops (requires a Web cam at the student side and is very bandwidth intensive), and records the entire class session for asynchronous playback.

Presentation of Materials

Most nurse educators are aware of presentation software such as PowerPoint and routinely use such applications in their courses. Yet, further clarification or explanation of content can be added by providing audio narration. Because these features are available as part of the presentation package, this solution can be distributed to multiple educators at low costs. Audio narration can be used to supplement traditional classes or in lieu of face-to-face meetings. When capturing the synchronized audio, typically instructors cannot pause or suspend the process. The resulting files can be converted to Web files for access via the Internet or, with the addition of other applications, converted to other Web-based formats.

Instead of using the audio narration contained within the presentation packages, screen recorders such as Camtasia (TechSmith Corporation, Okemos, MI) can also be used to provide audio narration of slide shows. The advantage in using screen recorders is that they usually allow the instructor to pause or suspend the recording. Similar to audio narration of static slides, screen recorders synchronize accompanying audio with the capture of the desktop screen display. These tools are particularly useful for demonstrating various software products such as spreadsheets and statistical software. Besides purchasing additional hardware such as headphones and Web cams, costs are incurred for site licensing, which prevents widespread distribution of this technology among instructors or learners.

Unfortunately, neither audio narration nor screen recorders can be used to capture live classes. Both of these technologies have higher learning curves and require additional training and technical support. Furthermore, instructors must be comfortable with teaching without live participant feedback or spontaneous commentaries. The use of videostreaming for live classes requires not only the videotaping itself by personnel, but the infrastructure to both encode, store, and deliver the final product.

Content Development Tools

Corporations and organizations use a fundamentally different approach to designing course material than colleges and universities. Academic institutions teach so many classes they have to mass produce any materials the instructor cares to put online.

Typically these would be PowerPoint presentations that the instructor might augment with an audio narration track. They are not interactive in nature except they allow the user to go back and forth to review whatever the instructor said earlier.

Corporations, on the other hand, have the financial resources to create highly interactive online course materials that can be placed into an LMS environment. They produce fewer courses, but more feature rich online courses since the cost of producing these online courses can easily offset the cost of hiring a face-to-face instructor and taking people out of production to take a course synchronously. The upfront costs for this kind of development, however, can be daunting. In the university environment the instructor can take an existing PowerPoint template and add content. After narrating within PowerPoint, the instructor can then post it on the course management system as an external link. This solution typically requires only the instructor. However, highly interactive course material that branches on specific answers and allows the student to move around the course in a nonlinear fashion takes significant effort and expense. This is typically well beyond the resources of a university, but often well within the resources of a corporation or organization that otherwise can be overwhelmed with the expense of securing a part-time instructor to teach a specific topic. Developing highly interactive courses requires a variety of skills including a subject matter expert (SME) who is knowledgeable about what computers can and cannot do in the area of instruction; an instructional designer who will develop the overall look and feel and navigation for the course; a graphics designer who will put in the graphics needed inside the course and the graphics that will make the course look professional; and a software programmer who will write the computer code that displays the content, deals with the interactive logic, and posts the data to the LMS. Of course, once the up-front time for developing the course has been paid for, the course requires no additional financial resources as long as no changes are required. Typically this approach works best in courses with highly stable course content over time. There is clearly a major software investment to develop course content in this environment. The graphics designer will need a graphics program to create the images and graphics the SME will want within the course. Products like Adobe Photoshop and Adobe Illustrator are expensive and not trivial to use, but most likely the graphics designer already has access to and knowledge about these applications.

Assembling the course requires a programming language and programming tools. Thankfully there are a number of relatively easy-to-use and powerful products available on the market today. The decision as to where this course will be hosted and whether it will be accessible via the Web (albeit through a password-protection mechanism) will help decide what product the software programmer will use. Products that work well with the Web include Adobe Flash, Adobe Dreamweaver, Trivantis' Lectora, and the new Web product Webtora. Products like Microsoft FrontPage and Adobe GoLive have been discontinued but can still function quite well here if they are available.

A big concern in this environment is how to deal with streaming media (audio and video) that are part of a course. Until recently, if an instructor wanted to put video into a course the students would have to live with long download times or the media would have to be uploaded to a separate streaming server. Media servers are costly to maintain. A new innovation from Adobe allows for video stored in FLV (flash video) format to be streamed from any Web server. This means the video can now be stored with the content on the LMS saving the time and expense of maintaining a separate streaming media server.

Clinical Education

Two clinical educational activities that can be enhanced with Web-based tools are physical demonstrations and clinical logs. At first glance, it would seem easy to capture digital video for physical demonstrations such as assessment or clinical procedures. However, to produce quality digital video requires expensive equipment and a production crew to attend to audio levels, lightning, and postproduction editing. With the widespread availability of digital still cameras, an alternative is to capture still digital photos. If these photos are arranged and timed to display in sequence, a close approximation can be obtained. If programming support is available, digital movies using still photos can be created using other applications such as Flash (Adobe Systems Incorporated, San Jose, CA).

As can be seen here, the more sophisticated the technique, the more time, energy, and funds are needed to create electronic educational tools. Consideration must be given to achieving a balance between the expense of creating the learning activity and the benefits. Although Web-based formats offer the additional advantages of flexibility, accessibility, and the ability to view the materials as often as is necessary, these benefits may not outweigh the expense.

Another tool to support clinical education is an electronic clinical log. Clinical education of nurses can involve direct clinical supervision by preceptors especially for nurse practitioner students. Faculty members are responsible for student progression, evaluation, and attainment of course objectives but must collect data to document a learner's clinical experiences. Typically this involves on-site visits, discussions with preceptors, and paper logs. With these approaches there is significant delay in receiving information from the learner and clinical supervisor and in giving appropriate feedback. In addition, it is very difficult and time consuming to aggregate data for a given learner or across learners for a given term or rotation.

Electronic clinical logs offer an alternative for documenting the types of clinical experiences learners are involved in as part of their educational program. Desirable features of such logs include ease of use, Web entry of data, standardized data entry, flagging of selected records for review or comment, linking of repeated client encounters, creation of student portfolios, and customization of the fields to reflect various professional standards and differences in specialties. The ability to aggregate data and create reports or charts is valuable. Using a PDA to record encounters at the point of care allows the learner to upload to the database at a later time.

Educational institutions can opt to create their own clinical log or purchase a commercial product, such as Typhon's Student Tracking Systems (Typhon Group Health care Solutions, Metairie, LA). Gordon and colleagues[10] discuss the advantages and disadvantages of both approaches. Depending on the size of the nursing program, commercial products may be cost prohibited and do require customization. On the other hand, creating an electronic clinical log requires considerable computer programming expertise.

Types of analyses that can be obtained from electronic clinical logs are demonstrated by Trangenstein and colleagues.[11] More than 85,000 records of 200 advanced practice nursing students in six different specialties in the span of 1 year were studied. Results obtained compared encounter times, number of encounters, types of clients seen, and services provided. Overall data showed that students definitely gained clinical experience and confidence as they progressed in their academic program.

SUMMARY

Never before has there been such a wide range of electronic educational tools available to enhance learning in nursing, automate some of the more routine tasks associated with a course, or to facilitate greater efficiency in using valuable face-to-face time. The challenge for nurse educators is to assimilate the knowledge and expertise to understand and appropriately use these electronic educational tools. This article attempts to acquaint nurse educators with the variety of choices available and common issues associated with their adoption.

While this article treated the available tools as discrete applications, more frequently software programs are incorporating an assortment of these tools. As a general rule, the more simultaneous, natural interaction the learning activity requires, the more expensive (in terms of time, energy, and funding) is the solution. For those nurse educators who are willing to change the way they teach, there is an abundance of Web-based educational tools available.

Web-based formats offer the advantages of allowing the learner to view course materials when they choose, from anywhere (as long as there is an Internet connection, preferably high speed) and as often as they want. Ill-conceived adoption of one or more of these tools is ineffective and can have the unintended consequence of frustrating educators by increasing time spent on designing and delivering instruction. If nurse educators feel that incorporation of these tools into current instruction activities requires too much effort, change is unlikely.

New Web-based educational tools will continue to be developed and nurse educators cannot afford to be left behind. For example, work has begun on using peer-to-peer networks to enable multimedia streaming over the Internet.[12] The challenge for nurse educators is to assimilate the knowledge and expertise to understand and appropriately use these electronic educational tools. Matching the appropriate solution to the proposed education activity is critical and may require support from others such as instructional designers and network technicians. Based on Morgan's study,[9] as instructors increase their awareness of possible solutions, they are likely to begin to restructure their courses and change the way they teach as they discover new ways to use an electronic educational toolkit.

ACKNOWLEDGMENT

The author acknowledges the contributions of Dr. Jeffry Gordon, Vanderbilt University, to the revision of this manuscript.

REFERENCES

1. Feretic E. Never too old. Beyond computing 2000. Available at: http://www.datacards.com/kdm/kdm37613.htm.
2. Chickering AW, Gamson ZF. Seven principles for good practice in undergraduate education. The American Association for Higher Education Bulletin 1987;39:3–7.
3. EduTools. EduTools Homepage. Available at: http://www.edutools.info/index.jsp?pj=1. Accessed March 25, 2008.
4. Chism N. Handbook for instructors on the use of electronic class discussion. Office of Faculty and TA Development, The Ohio State University. Available at: http://ftad.osu.edu/Publications/elecdisc/pages/index.htm. Accessed March 27, 2008.
5. Murphy KL, Collins MP. Development of communication conventions in instructional electronic chats. Journal of Distance Education 1998;12(1/2):177–200. Available at: http://disted.tamu.edu/aera97a.htm. Accessed March 30, 2008.
6. Smith CW. Synchronous discussion in online courses: a pedagogical strategy for taming the chat beast. Learning Circuits 2006; (July). Available at: http://www.learningcircuits.org/2006/July/smith.htm. Accessed March 27, 2008.
7. Netlingo. The list of chat acronyms & text message shorthand. Available at: http://www.netlingo.com/emailsh.cfm. Accessed March 30, 2008.

8. Windweaver TM. Recommended emoticons for email communication. Available at: http://www.windweaver.com/emoticon.htm. Accessed March 30, 2008.

9. Morgan G. Faculty use of course management systems. Educause Center for Applied Research 2003; (May). Available at: http://www.educause.edu/ir/library/pdf/ERS0302/ekf0302.pdf. Accessed March 26, 2008.

10. Gordon JS, McNew R, Trangenstein P. The development of an online clinical log for advanced practice nursing students: a case study. In: Kuhn KA, Warren JR, Leong T-Y, editors. MedInfo 2007. Amsterdam: IOS Press; 2007. p. 1432–6.

11. Trangenstein P, Weiner E, Gordon J, et al. Data mining results from an electronic clinical log for nurse practitioner students. In: Kuhn KA, Warren JR, Leong T-Y, editors. MedInfo 2007. Amsterdam: IOS Press; 2007. p. 1387–91.

12. VUCast. Vanderbilt engineer wins NSF award for innovative internet system. Vanderbilt University: February 15, 2007. Available at: http://www.vanderbilt.edu/news/releases/2007/2/15/vanderbilt-engineer-wins-nsf-award-for-innovative-internet-system. Accessed March 31, 2008.

Strategies for Success in Online Learning

Shirley W. Cantrell, PhD, RN, Patricia O'Leary, DSN, RN, COI,
Karen S. Ward, PhD, RN, COI*

KEYWORDS

• Nursing education • Distance education
• Educational technology

More and more nurses are finding themselves back in school; some as students, some as part-time or adjunct faculty members, and many seeking to obtain additional credentials. Nurses with expertise in a clinical specialty are highly valued as potential educators to assist with producing additional nursing graduates. Whether as a learner or a teacher or, sometimes, both, nurses frequently become involved with online educational delivery. Exploring ways to make online learning successful is important for anyone contemplating an entry into this educational option.

THE LEARNERS

Today, many nurses are experiencing pressure to advance their careers. Sometimes this pressure is coming from an employer, either to obtain a new position or to retain one already held. Just as frequently, this pressure to enhance credentials by returning to academia comes from within. The escalating demands for additional knowledge and skills affects nurses at all levels of the profession. In spite of the well-documented nursing shortage, or perhaps because of it, health care facilities are expecting a great deal from their nurses. Studies have shown that the more education nurses have, the better the outcomes for their patients.[1] Thus, licensed practical nurses (LPNs) are returning to school for degrees that allow them to practice as registered nurses (RNs). Diploma or associate degree–prepared RNs return to pursue their bachelor's degrees (BSN) and those with a BSN find themselves seeking masters (MSN) and doctoral degrees (PhD, EdD, DSN, DNP, and so forth).

Today's fast-paced lifestyle, decreased funding for physical facilities, and advanced technology have all added to the shift from classroom learning to online learning.[2] Along with the demand for additional education, most nurses are carrying heavy loads at work and at home. As a result of the nursing shortage, they are asked, and often expected, to take on even more overtime hours. At home, they are caring for children, parents, and frequently both. Despite high motivation to expand their academic

Box 81, School of Nursing, Middle Tennessee State University, Murfreesboro, TN 37132, USA
* Corresponding author.
E-mail address: kward@mtsu.edu (K.S. Ward).

Nurs Clin N Am 43 (2008) 547–555
doi:10.1016/j.cnur.2008.06.003
0029-6465/08/$ – see front matter © 2008 Elsevier Inc. All rights reserved.

nursing.theclinics.com

credentials, it is often difficult to find a way to take care of their obligations and get to class often enough to succeed in their courses.

The rapid expansion of online education has certainly offered an attractive mechanism to these highly motivated but "swamped with obligations" individuals. Being able to attend class on their own schedules is extremely appealing. Online learning also has the advantages of eliminating travel time and parking problems. There is no need for childcare or other sitter services because the student never needs to leave the house; all that is required is a computer and Internet access. Other benefits identified for online courses are the professional development and accountability for nurses, promoting lifelong, self-directed learning and the ability to reach a very diverse student population.[3] Online courses offer the advantage of more independent and interactive learning as well as more individualized learning experiences (**Box 1**).[4] Many nursing programs have developed online versions for some portion of their student population. Although fewer programs exist for initial licensure students, programs for RNs returning for their BSN or MSN are plentiful. During the academic year of 1994 to 1995, there were 753,640 students in distance education; in the academic year 2000 to 2001, the numbers jumped to over 3,077,000.[5]

THE EDUCATORS

Many factors contribute to the shortage of nursing faculty. On average, schools of nursing do not pay as well as clinical facilities. To teach, nurses must have advanced degrees and the percentage of nurses with these degrees is small. Findings from the 2004 National Sample Survey of Registered Nurses out of the Department of Health

---

Box 1
Benefits to online learning

✔ Does not require physical attendance

✔ Courses available 24/7

✔ Flexible scheduling

✔ Can access courses from any location (home, work, traveling)

✔ Self-paced workload

✔ Self-directed learning

✔ Multiple learning styles accommodated

✔ More individualized learning experiences

✔ Eliminates travel time

✔ Childcare and other sitter services unnecessary

✔ Decreases or eliminates costs such as parking and fuel

✔ Cultivates greater student interaction and collaboration

✔ Fosters greater student-instructor communication

✔ Enhances computer and Internet skills

✔ Retention of material as good as standard classroom

✔ Promotes professional development and accountability

✔ Reaches diverse student population

and Human Services revealed that only 12% of nurses have a Master's Degree and even fewer, a mere 0.8% hold a docorate (http://bhpr.hrsa.gov/healthworkforce/rnsurvey04). However, the overriding problem is that there is a severe shortage of nurses in general. The sad truth is that unless there are more nursing faculty, there cannot be more nurses; and without more nurses, more nursing faculty cannot be produced. This circular situation is a very difficult one. Schools of nursing are trying to address it in part by recruiting clinical experts for part-time or adjunct positions.

Despite the generally low salaries paid to these individuals, RNs who wonder if a future academic career is something they would enjoy often decide that the experience is worth their time, even with the small monetary reward. Nursing graduate students often accept graduate assistantships that involve teaching. These teaching assistant (TA) positions are often a good way for the student to receive paid tuition and a small stipend while taking classes.

Just like a potential student, the RN considering a teaching role may want to become involved in the online environment. And, like the student, the educator must decide if there is a fit with that format. Certainly there are similar trade-offs for the instructor as there are for the student and determining up-front whether online education will work is equally important.

GENERAL GUIDELINES

Before entering into a relationship with any educational endeavor, it pays to investigate and evaluate what is offered by different institutions. Especially with the mushrooming of online programs, it is crucial to make sure that the school is completely legitimate.[6] Potential students should look for evidence of accreditation through one of the two accrediting bodies for schools of nursing: the American Association of Colleges of Nursing-affiliated Commission on Collegiate Nursing Education (www.aacn.nche.edu) and the National League for Nursing Accrediting Commission (www.nlnac.org). Find out if the school is approved by the appropriate state board. This can be verified through the National Council of State Boards of Nursing (www.ncsbn.org).

Applying to a school that has an existing nursing program with a long-established reputation is the most reliable way to assure yourself that you are about to take courses or teach at a reputable institution, whether it is an online or on campus program. Companies have been created to offer degrees online in a number of disciplines. With the nursing shortage, they are adding nursing or related degrees to the list. Be very cautious before investing in such a program.

Other important characteristics are discussed in the following sections. As nurses consider whether or not to become involved with a specific academic institution, it is helpful to consider these factors. Individuals will have differing opinions as to which program best meets his or her needs, so it is important to ask questions directly at the institution being considered.

Flexibility

Most programs that offer online learning do so to provide flexibility in class attendance, giving students a choice in both time and location. Apart from this obvious advantage, there are other aspects of flexibility to look for in a program. RNs may not have to complete every required general education course before they begin nursing classes. To argue that they must have the content in an American History class before they take Community Health Nursing, for example, seems indefensible, especially since they have already passed the nursing licensure examination. For the same reason, they are frequently allowed to take the required nursing courses in the order that works best for them.

Another way flexibility can be demonstrated is when the program is self-paced. Students can take as many or as few courses as they wish. This allows them to complete the program in a time period that works best for them. It is very important that each student receive good advisement on the choice of how many courses to take at one time. Taking too few may lead to frustration with how long the program takes and taking too many may cause the student to feel overwhelmed and be unsuccessful. It is the student's choice, but an educated choice must be made.

Providing a Personal Touch

One of the biggest fears that online students voice is that they will not have enough help from faculty. Having online instructors who are available to students is extremely important. Students need to feel free to call or e-mail their instructors and to hear back from them in a timely manner. Some programs have standards regarding how quickly instructors will respond. While these standards provide guidelines and make expectations known to both faculty and students, they may not be necessary if the students are kept informed by the course instructor so that they know what to expect. Whether teaching or learning online, timeliness is important for all communications.

One way of welcoming students to a course is when instructors send students an e-mail or letter through regular mail before the start of class. When students get such correspondence, they are encouraged that their instructor is interested and eager to have them in class. Creating an "office" on one of the discussion boards is a helpful tool for online students and faculty alike. By having students ask general questions about the course in this public forum, the instructor's answer is also public and saves the instructor from having to answer numerous times. Another way to give the whole class helpful information is to have a list of frequently asked questions derived from previous classes and issues that were unclear to previous students.

Most students new to online learning are amazed at how well they get to know their classmates. Instructors are also taken by surprise when they realize that they know their online students better than those in traditional classrooms. This occurs for a variety of reasons, but seems to be a consistent finding in online courses. Building a community of learners is very important and a key component of online education. RNs tend to respond very well to expectations involving interaction on discussion boards. Student discussions and questions stimulate other classmates to think. Their comments are more open and students are less inhibited about speaking their thoughts or challenging others' comments when interacting via computer as opposed to speaking up in class. Some students are too timid to speak in an on-ground class, but not in an online course, and this is one real advantage. A strategy that often works with students who do not participate in discussion is to e-mail them privately and encourage them to participate. Once students do get involved in the discussion, providing positive feedback helps them to feel successful and thus continue interaction. Some faculty resort to providing actual credit for online class participation.

Most online course formats provide a feature where the student can create a "home page." Using this option as part of the course expectations is an important way to engage students with each other. Requiring a picture as part of the page allows students to get to know their classmates so that they might recognize them on the street (if they are ever on the same street!). Students' comments and faculty feedback indicate that they enjoy this assignment because they are able to put a face with the name on the discussion board or in a chat room.

Computer Guidance

Many students and faculty return to school after a number of years feeling that they lack computer skills. Time concern is exacerbated by the stress of having to deal with technology problems, learning new online software, and learning a large amount of new material at the same time.[7] According to Halstead and Coudret[8] "it can be guaranteed that technical issues will develop during teaching of the online course" (page 5). In fact, taking an online course does not require a depth of computer knowledge. For the most part, as long as someone can use e-mail, knows how to use a word processor, and is able to attach a document to e-mail, the mechanics of an online course an be mastered. Student and faculty support in the form of orientation to technology, learning resources, and student services should be in place before starting online courses.[7] When they do experience problems, students often become a resource for each other as they share their experiences and solutions.[9] As adult learners they bring experience-based insights and viewpoints about computers and nursing in general.[10]

Programs can create a list of basic computer requirements, both hardware and software, that will be needed to be able to easily navigate the courses. When faculty provide this information before the start of the program, participants purchase what they do not already have and feel more fully prepared. Links to a help desk and similar resources, such as the library and university writing center, should be expected in online courses.

Many times students or faculty who live in rural areas must access their courses using a dial-up Internet connection. Although it is certainly possible to participate in courses that way, it can produce significant frustration, so it is useful to search out a high-speed option. Accessing the Internet at places of employment solves this problem for many in online education. Libraries provide another viable alternative.

One strategy that has worked well in helping students navigate a course is the creation of a Scavenger Hunt as a first assignment. For the "hunt," each student must "roam" around the course and find things that the instructor has listed. This forces them to overcome their fear of clicking on all the buttons and finding out what is contained in the course. In the scavenger hunt, students are required to use the tools they will be using during the course such as course e-mail, discussion forums, and the "drop box" for submitting assignments. This helps to decrease students' anxiety about the online environment, especially the student who is weak in computer skills. Students report that they like this assignment very much and that it introduces them to the course in a very user-friendly way. Faculty find that after such an assignment, students ask fewer basic questions about course details.

Well-Constructed Courses

Courses should be user friendly, logically structured, and easy to navigate (**Box 2**). Careful communication is needed when there is no face-to-face contact between faculty and students; expectations must be very clear.[8] Assignments need to be understandable, with clear grading policies. Faculty need to make sure the site is designed to accommodate a range of users from the skilled to not so skilled.[7] Billings[7] identified seven principles of good practice in education via online courses: active learning, time on task, collaboration with peers, interaction with faculty, rich and rapid feedback, high expectations, and respect for diversity.

Use of a variety of strategies that address a diverse range of learning styles (visual, auditory, kinesthetic) is important. Multiple assessment strategies are preferred over a singular approach, such as tests. If given the opportunity to preview courses before deciding on a program, students should look for this user-friendly environment.

Box 2
Attributes of user-friendly online courses

☑ Faculty available to answer questions in timely fashion

☑ Variety of mechanisms employed for students and faculty to get to know one another (homepage, discussion boards, chat rooms)

☑ Strategies to help students become comfortable with course are evident (scavenger hunt, practice tests, and so forth)

☑ Testing is online and offered over many time frames

☑ Course logically structured and easy to navigate

☑ Course expectations outlined and clear

☑ Grading policies posted and understandable

☑ Rich and rapid feedback provided students on assignments, course activities

☑ Site designed to accommodate computer users at many skill levels

☑ Variety of teaching strategies to accommodate a diverse range of learning styles

The amount and quality of interactivity in an online course has been identified by students and faculty as one of the most important aspects to successful online learning.[3,5] Instructor unfamiliarity with technology can make it very difficult to promote online interactivity. Faculty should be comfortable in using all technological tools available in the course format, and then use these activities to encourage critical and reflective thinking thereby engaging students.[5]

Various types of interactions have been identified by online faculty as very beneficial to learning. These include learner-instructor interactions, learner-learner interactions, and learner-content interactions.[5] Students are encouraged to read other students' postings even if they are not responding to each one. Variations in amount and type of interaction may reflect difference in personality and learning styles, not necessarily the amount of learning.

PowerPoint presentations are commonly used in online courses. It is important to include more than words in the presentations. The use of pictures, graphs, Web sites, and audio are all strategies that faculty can use to enhance the "lecture" experience. However, pictures and audio take longer to open especially for the student who has a slower computer or Internet connection. Converting a PowerPoint file into a compressed program such as Impatica is very helpful. These files are typically 95% smaller than normal PowerPoint HTML files. Students are able to open the PowerPoint presentations without any difficulty and do not need to worry about having PowerPoint software on their computer when such a program is used.

Grading policies and clear expectations regarding all assignments are essential. Particularly with discussion forums, this is very important. Using a rubric system for grading is one way is to accomplish clarity. Rubrics serve to alert the student to what is expected for each grade and to assist other faculty who might teach the course at a later time in knowing how to grade each student (**Box 3** for an example).

A timed practice test is a strategy that helps decrease anxiety for those who have never taken a timed test online. Another plan that works well in regard to testing is making the tests available for several days during the week, including weekend and week days. This approach helps accommodate the students' work and personal schedules. Making a test available for part of 1 day (ie, a 4-hour time period) or

---

Box 3
Example of an assignment grading rubric

1 Point

    Minimal response to the module question or minimal response to classmate's posting (ie, I agree with your comments…). Shows no engagement in the discussion forum.

2 points

    Makes 2 or more postings responding to the question. However, the postings are not substantial enough to stimulate further class discussion. Shows some engagement in the discussion.

3 points

    3 or more postings that fully address the module question/student's comments, Postings stimulate follow-up posting by classmates. Shows full engagement in the discussion forum.

---

allowing only one 24-hour day for test completion does not work well and tends to negate the desired flexibility of an online course. A primary goal of online programming is flexibility. Creating too small a window for testing eliminates some of the much-prized flexibility. Testing itself is stress provoking and issues of test submission can intensify the process.

ONGOING EVALUATION

Opportunities to voice opinions about the online learning process in general, as well as their specific courses, is something students value. Getting this ongoing feedback from students is important to maintaining a successful program. Uppermost in their thoughts is the flexibility that the online environment offers. They are able to work at home and at their own pace, at a time that is convenient for them. They mention that "travel time and expense are obsolete," and students see that as a big advantage to online learning. These comments from students appear consistently in online course evaluations across a variety of disciplines.[3,4,7–9]

    Advice that students and faculty might offer others interested in this educational option generally center around two major themes: concern regarding technology problems and issues regarding the learning process itself. One way to approach the technology concern is to stay in contact with the instructor. For example, more often than not, if the system is down or some other connection problem exists, the instructor is experiencing the same situation and will work to remedy it. Students new to the online process need to be very self-motivated and willing to create their own learning times. Procrastination is a major barrier to good online learning. With self-paced, flexible scheduling, things can pile up very quickly. Often the best plan is to access the course for a short time every day, rather than opting for a large block of time less frequently. That way, if computer problems occur when logging on, the next day offers an opportunity for quick recovery. Students consistently recommend finding a way to keep up with due dates in their online courses. One suggestion is to make a calendar on a dry-erase board, where it is seen everyday, and assignments or tests are clearly visible. Both faculty and students need to be aware that online courses will not make their workload less, just more flexible. In fact, many will find they spend more time with their online courses than they do with traditional courses.

    Many faculty members express a concern that students may not learn as much in an online course as compared with an on-ground course. Cramer and colleagues[11] indicated that students in an online class actually used the virtual lecture hall more frequently, for longer periods of time, and made better grades. The personality and learning styles of students who take online courses may also contribute to the comfort level with online learning which allows these students to learn at least as much as the on ground classes.

Teaching online can be a bit intimidating for faculty new to the experience. Faculty inexperienced with online teaching will require a lot of technical support especially in the initial development of courses,[4,5] when a significant amount time is required for the development of online courses.[3,10] Design experts have estimated that it takes about 10 hours of preparation for each hour of traditional class time.[3] Online teaching is more than just putting your PowerPoint slides on the Web. Many faculty members have tried to just translate their traditional lectures rather than transform the course.[5] Faculty members need workshops in Web instruction and design as well as orientation to technology before they begin teaching online classes. They need ongoing tech support as well as workload adjustment, rewards, and recognition.[7]

SUMMARY

In today's fast paced and rapidly changing health care environment, nurses often want to participate in online learning, a very attractive and frequently chosen option that facilitates acquisition of more advanced degrees. It is also a great option for part-time teaching. Faculty teaching in the online environment should create the most comfortable atmosphere possible for returning students. Students gain a lot by having more flexibility in course offerings that allow them to achieve their educational goals. With explicit expectations in the online learning environment, individuals involved in the process can achieve success. Goals are met for students and faculty alike through a flexible avenue providing choices in time and location unavailable until the advent of this learning format.

REFERENCES

1. Aiken LH, Clarke SP, Cheung RB, et al. Educational levels of hospital nurses and surgical patient mortality. JAMA 2003;390(12):1617–23.
2. Karber DJ. Comparisons and contrasts in traditional versus on-line teaching in management. Higher Education in Europe 2002;XXVI(4):533–6.
3. Bentley G, Cook P, Davis K, et al. RN to BSN program transition from traditional to online delivery. Nurse Educ 2003;28(3):121–6.
4. Lashley M. Teaching health assessment in the virtual classroom. J Nurs Educ 2005;44(8):348–50.
5. Su B, Bonk CJ, Magjuka RJ, et al. The importance of interaction in Web-based education: a program-level case study of online MBA courses. Journal of Interactive Online Learning 2005;4(1):1–19.
6. Trossman S. Issues up close. American Nurse Today 2007;2(9):37–8.
7. Billings DM. A framework for assessing outcomes and practices in Web-based courses in nursing. J Nurs Educ 2000;39(2):60–7.
8. Halstead JA, Coudret NA. Implementing Web-based instruction in a baccalaureate nursing program. 2006. Available at: http://www.ihets.org/archive/progserv_arc/education_arc/faculty_papers_c. Accessed October 7, 2006.
9. Cartwright J. Lessons learned: using asynchronous computer-mediated conferencing to facilitate group discussion. J Nurs Educ 2000;39(2):87–90.

10. Shovein J, Huston C, Fox S, et al. Challenging traditional teaching and learning paradigms: online learning and emancipatory teaching. Nurs Educ Perspect 2005;26(6):340–3.
11. Cramer KM, Collins K, Snider D, et al. Virtual lecture hall for in class and online sections: a comparison of utilization, perceptions, and benefits. Journal of Research on Technology in Education 2006;38(4):371–81.

Doctoral Education from a Distance

Judith A. Effken, PhD, RN, FACMI, FAAN

KEYWORDS

- Doctoral education • Distance education • Online education
- Nursing education

Today we are facing what may be the most severe nursing shortage in our history—and one that has no end in sight. Although the population continues to increase and baby boomers age, adding to the strain on our health care systems, many nursing faculty are approaching retirement.[1] Nursing programs are attempting to increase the number of nursing graduates they produce, but are limited, in part, by the number of qualified, doctorally prepared faculty available. In 2005 and 2006, 88,000 (1 of every 3) qualified applicants to nursing education programs were rejected because of lack of capacity. Even with the addition of 150 new registered nurse programs in 2005 and 2006, overall enrollment growth actually declined from 3% in 2005 to 1.5% in 2006. The selectivity of nursing programs significantly exceeds that of other United States undergraduate programs, with 54% of 4-year college nursing programs admitting less than half their applicants in 2006, compared with 35% for United States 4-year colleges in general.[2]

Despite the increase in the number of nursing doctoral programs in the United States, until recently the number of PhD graduates has not increased significantly. In 2007, although enrollment increased by 6.3% (231 students) to a total of 3927 students, the number of graduates increased by only 1.4% (6 students).[3] Attrition rates in doctoral programs have been reported as high as 50%.[1,4] As a result, most doctoral programs graduate only a few students each year.

According to American Association of Colleges of Nursing statistics, nurses who enter doctoral programs often do so late in their careers; as a result, the average age of new nursing PhDs is 46, which is much older than the average new PhD in other fields (32–35). This age difference means that the doctorally prepared nurses we are producing have much less career time to develop a research program or teach.[1]

Historically, doctoral education has used an apprenticeship model in which students study intensively with faculty mentors to gain the knowledge, skills, and lore needed to conduct independent research. This model is still the norm in most of the sciences—and many assume that it is also the norm for nursing doctoral

The University of Arizona College of Nursing, 1305 North Martin, PO Box 210203, Tucson, AZ 85721-0203, USA
E-mail address: jeffken@nursing.arizona.edu

Nurs Clin N Am 43 (2008) 557–566
doi:10.1016/j.cnur.2008.06.007
0029-6465/08/$ – see front matter © 2008 Elsevier Inc. All rights reserved.

nursing.theclinics.com

education. However, the apprenticeship model has limited our ability to attract nurses to doctoral education for several reasons:

Nurses who may aspire to doctoral education are nearly always employed, either as faculty, staff, or administrators, and frequently cannot or do not want to leave that employment.

Nurses have family responsibilities that may preclude their moving to engage in full-time, on-campus study that an apprenticeship model requires.

Geography too can be a barrier. For example, The University of Arizona has had a well-regarded doctoral program for many years, but its location in southern Arizona has made access difficult for students. Some commuting students have driven many miles to come to campus; some have even flown. Others have actually moved to study here in Tucson. Still, the number of students who graduated as PhDs remained low (perhaps three to five per year), and the vast majority attended on a part-time basis, which meant that their education took longer and they were older on graduating with limited time remaining in which to conduct research or teach. Outside of class time, these part-time students spent little time on campus with faculty so, to a great extent, the apprenticeship model of doctoral education was, for most students, a myth. Only a few students (often international students) were actually on campus full time and engaged in faculty research as graduate research assistants or associates.

As nurse educators were pushed to expand capacity, they began to look at other models of delivering doctoral education. Could educators bring doctoral education to students rather than expecting them to come to campus? Could students be provided with the needed research mentorship at a distance?

For faculty at The University of Arizona, the gauntlet was thrown down by the Arizona Board of Regents in 2003, who challenged the three state-funded schools of nursing to double their enrollments by 2008. As the only doctoral program in Arizona at that time, we determined to increase not only our baccalaureate graduates, but also our PhD graduates. Doing so would mean determining how we could make doctoral education more accessible to nurses.[5]

USING TECHNOLOGY TO DELIVER EDUCATION: INITIAL EFFORTS

Distance education has a long history, initially as correspondence courses in which students worked largely independently, reading and then submitting assignments to the instructor by mail. In the past 10 to 15 years, however, technology has made other options for delivering distance education available, such as television and online delivery. Malone College and Duquesne University began offering their nursing PhD programs online in 1997. The University of Arizona's online nursing PhD program, which began in 2003, was the first at a research-extensive university. Other online PhD programs have followed quickly (eg, University of Utah, University of Colorado at Denver and Health Sciences, Northern Colorado University, Oregon Health Sciences University, Vanderbilt University, Medical College of South Carolina, University of Wisconsin-Milwaukee, University of Kansas, University of Hawaii, Rutgers University, and so forth).

At the University of Arizona, before the Board of Regents' challenge, we had already begun to televise some graduate courses to a second site in Phoenix by way of the Arizona Telemedicine Program's telecommunication network. Because some of our students lived in the Phoenix metropolitan area, this made perfect sense. Students could choose either to come to campus or to attend class from the Phoenix site. This technology had several limitations, however. First, from a teaching perspective, it was challenging to engage students at the Phoenix site in discussions with the students in the classroom. Second, our ability to provide education by this method was limited to Arizona—and realistically just to this second site in Phoenix. We also had begun to deliver part of our master's courses online—initially in a hybrid format in which part of the course was online and part was face-to-face. A few instructors had moved to a fully online model.

At a faculty retreat, we reflected on what we valued in our current doctoral program and what might be improved. After discussing the relative strengths and limitations of televised and online delivery modes, we opted for a fully online program. We believed that this technology would best allow us to increase nurses' access to doctoral education and that it would be more engaging as well.

Most distributed nursing doctoral programs across the country use some combination of online and face-to-face instruction. In general, most course work is online with content provided in various formats (video, text, demonstration) and subsequent asynchronous discussions or synchronous interactive video or chat sessions. The University of Utah uses regularly scheduled interactive video sessions in which students participate in synchronous discussions. Most programs include some amount of on-campus time (7–14 days, typically) in which students are oriented to the program and software, participate in varied research experiences (or clinical experiences, in the case of the Doctorate of Nursing Practice [DNP]), and are socialized into doctoral study and the program itself. Some online doctoral programs require students to come to campus more frequently, and some course content may also be provided during this face-to-face time.

When we first embarked on this journey, many of us were skeptical. Given the need for extensive individual mentoring, how could doctoral education possibly be provided effectively at a distance? We have come to recognize, however, that doctoral education may be the most amenable level for distance education because the online format demands that students have a high degree of self-motivation. Typically, the doctoral students we admit have more clearly defined educational goals and a history of successful academic study.

THE COMMUNITY OF INQUIRY MODEL

One of the more popular contemporary models for online education is that of Community of Inquiry (**Fig. 1**).[6] Building an effective learning community online has been a major concern because of the preponderance of asynchronous interaction and the potential for isolation. Considerable evidence now exists that such a community

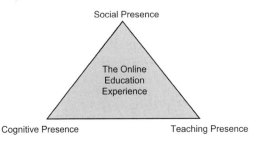

Fig. 1. The community of inquiry.

can be built successfully online,[7,8] although as Garrison and colleagues[6] point out, doing so is not trivial. A sense of community has been shown to be linked with students' perceived learning, if not with their actual learning outcomes,[9,10] and perceived learning is associated with student retention and progression (see **Fig. 1**).[11]

The Community of Inquiry model makes intuitive sense for distance doctoral programs because these programs are explicitly aimed at scholarly inquiry (research in the case of the PhD and practice inquiry in the case of the DNP). Moreover, doctoral students typically share common goals and interests with faculty and with each other, both of which are necessary for community building.[6] For PhD students, it is expected that students and faculty together work to build nursing science, with students' research typically building on that of the faculty with whom they are working.

Social Presence

Social presence has been defined as the degree to which faculty and students are able to project their unique personal characteristics so that they are viewed as real people. Distance doctoral programs present unique challenges to creating social presence because so much of the interaction is text-based. As a result, nonverbal information, such as facial expressions and voice tones, is not available. Faculty can enhance social presence by providing timely responses to student questions and maintaining faculty visibility in group discussions. Faculty also can build social presence by contributing their own experiential knowledge and research data to the discussion.

In our program, we begin building social presence as soon as students are admitted to the program. Newly admitted students are encouraged to get acquainted by e-mail. By the time they come to their first Research Intensive Summer Experience (just before their first semester in the program), they already have begun to make friends. Because they progress through core content as cohorts, these students soon know each other very well indeed. Rumors and news travel as fast by the Internet as in our hallways. Still, there is a time (usually about mid-spring) when a sense of isolation emerges among students and faculty alike. To counter that, we strongly encourage our students to attend the Western Institute of Nursing Research Conference and have been able to offer them partial financial support for this activity. Students are encouraged to present posters or give podium presentations related to their research. Our faculty often uses this conference time to hold face-to-face class sessions. Faculty members also meet with their advisees, and the College of Nursing holds a reception for students, alumni, and faculty. This experience provides a "booster shot" that renews energy and community.

Cognitive Presence

Cognitive presence has been defined as the extent to which a group of students and faculty together can construct meaning through sustained communication. Garrison and colleagues[6] describe cognitive presence as a cycle of inquiry in which students move from understanding the problem or issue at hand, through exploring the issue more deeply, integrating new with previous knowledge, and finally applying the concepts themselves. Like others, we have found the early stages of inquiry easier to facilitate, but doing so requires engaging students in interesting, complex problems (sometimes called challenges). The latter stages (synthesis and application), which require that students spend more time on reflection and "connecting the dots" among disparate content, are more difficult, particularly for distance students who are carrying out multiple roles (student, employee, parent, caregiver). In many cases, it is the student's synthesis seminar, individual preparation for the comprehensive examination, or dissertation effort in which the necessary integration finally occurs because in each of these efforts, students must explicitly focus on review and integration. This is when we most often observe students having "aha!" moments in which they suddenly realize how concepts learned in the philosophy of science have real and practical importance for their own areas of study and the methods they will use to answer their research questions.

Teaching Presence

Teaching presence refers to the faculty role in designing the educational experience, setting and communicating goals, and facilitating discussion and learning. Courses taught face-to-face need to be substantially, if not totally, redesigned for online delivery. We can say with a degree of confidence that any course can be taught online, but that different techniques and strategies are needed than in the classroom. We have had the good fortune and funding to be able to give faculty release time to rethink how they would teach their courses online. In addition, we have been fortunate to have a technology team, including an instructional designer, to help with the transition. Both have been extremely valuable. Research tells us that students recall little from lectures, so perhaps it is a benefit of distance learning that teachers lecture less and, when they do, the lectures are in a format that can be replayed by students for better retention. Teaching presence also includes designing discussions and activities that achieve the desired learning outcomes. Perhaps one of the more difficult transitions for faculty is making the shift from presenter to facilitator. Although there are many helpful books on how to facilitate online discussions, instructors eventually must determine for themselves when and how to participate in the discussions. Sometimes I have to sit on my hands to avoid prematurely responding to student comments and thereby inhibiting student discussion and discovery. Still, if students clearly are going down a wrong path, it is essential for faculty to intervene quickly.

TECHNOLOGIES TO SUPPORT DOCTORAL EDUCATION AT A DISTANCE

There are several course management systems that allow faculty to create and manage course content and delivery. These typically include the ability to store text-based or video-based content and support asynchronous discussion, synchronous chat, and quizzes. Initially we investigated a course management system designed not for students but for business that would have allowed us to recreate the physical layout of the College of Nursing. The approach was appealing visually and theoretically, but proved to be too expensive. Whether navigation in the environment would have enhanced students' experience or simply added a layer of complexity to their navigation remains an open question.

To supplement the basic toolsets available in course management systems, there are an increasing number of interactive videoconferencing tools that facilitate synchronous communication. Current bandwidth limitations may necessitate the use of additional audio technology (either telephone or computer based, such as Skype) to realize the benefits of videoconferencing. Various screen-capturing software applications can be used by faculty to demonstrate the use of various technologies—or simply to explain a conceptual model by recording their computer activity with simultaneous narration.

One of the newest technologies to support communities of inquiry in general and teaching presence specifically is asynchronous audio feedback using WAV files that instructors create and insert into discussion postings and papers. Ice and colleagues found that this kind of embedded audio feedback conveyed more nuances than text-based feedback, enhanced community and interaction, increased retention, and was associated with increased student satisfaction and perceptions that instructors cared more about students.[12]

Many educators are currently experimenting with the use of computer-based simulated environments or "virtual worlds" (eg, Second Life or Active Worlds) as instructional environments. Several universities, including ours, have purchased space in Second Life for faculty to experiment. These virtual worlds allow faculty to create, virtually, a specific environment that they want distance students to experience. Students and faculty create avatars that may or may not resemble themselves, but can move about and interact. Initially, virtual worlds supported only text-based interaction, but audio is now available also. Today's virtual worlds can support educational games, simulations, collaborative projects, and even embedded evaluation.

Virtual worlds can be exceedingly powerful, as in one educational example designed by a psychiatrist to demonstrate what it is like to be a paranoid schizophrenic. As my avatar moved through the virtual environment, the floor on which I walked appeared to melt away. When I attempted to read a virtual newspaper, threatening words seemed to jump off the page. Even more disturbing were the persistent negative messages.

We intend to use Second Life to replicate the United States–Mexico border for our Border Health students and also to create a kind of Socratic forum for students to work with their peers to prepare for the oral comprehensive examination. Such virtual worlds are labor intensive to build, and students' learning outcomes are only beginning to be reported. Still, given their potential to increase social presence, we can expect to see even more interest in these environments as more are developed and their effects on social, cognitive, and teaching presence are assessed.

CHALLENGES TO PROVIDING DOCTORAL EDUCATION AT A DISTANCE

Undoubtedly the most challenging part of providing doctoral education at a distance is research mentoring. Providing effective mentoring is a critical component of doctoral education. Students must learn not only the theory and methods needed for their research, but also the research lore that faculty can impart—lessons from the trenches, so to speak, on managing research teams, budgets, and schedules, working through Investigational Review Board regulations, research ethics, and so forth. Many programs use on-site research intensives to help bridge this gap. Some of our faculty have designed additional research experiences for their advisees during the research intensive, such as analyzing data from an ongoing study. Other faculty include distance students as members of their research teams. To facilitate mentoring at a distance, we created an electronically enhanced meeting room that allows interactive videoconferencing and a secure, encrypted server in which data can be safely shared by faculty researchers with their off-site research assistants. Still, students who are doing bench research may need to come to campus to access laboratory equipment and they are made aware of this prior to admission.

In reviews of National Research Service Award applications, the National Institute of Nursing Research (NINR) has challenged the amount and type of research mentoring that students in distance PhD programs receive. As we implement more rigorous and effective ways of mentoring, it will be necessary to demonstrate the effectiveness of these methods to external reviewers and NINR staff, and to other potential critics of distance education. As our graduates become established researchers and leaders, we expect some of these issues to diminish. Still, we need to enhance our research mentoring creatively and educate others in how this can and is being done effectively.

In the past, students often took their minor cognate in diverse fields (eg, psychology, sociology, anthropology), but these programs are frequently not available online. At The University of Arizona our students now often take nearly all their coursework within the College of Nursing. This practice clearly limits our students' opportunities for study to some degree.

A related challenge is being able to provide the breadth and depth of knowledge in several emphasis areas—particularly when major and minor cognates must be taken within the same program. This challenge has led us to implement several minor options (eg, Border Health, Workforce and Healthcare Delivery Environments, Gerontology, Informatics, Nursing Systems, and Rural Health). Maintaining a cadre of faculty who can teach not only core nursing science and research courses but also the content for these additional options is challenging. In addition, the number of students in a particular cognate may be low, necessitating independent studies, which clearly are expensive to provide.

Nationally, two responses to these challenges are worth noting: The Midwestern Big 10 universities have an agreement that allows students to take courses from faculty at any of their universities and have it count as a home course. This agreement is enabling students in, for example, informatics to study vocabulary issues with an expert at Iowa and human factors with an expert at Wisconsin. The Western Institute of Nursing has initiated a program, NEXus, that is aimed at a similar outcome. Five nursing PhD programs developed a set of shared cognates in which courses from various programs were approved as cognates or electives for students in any of the participating programs. Because there was no existing contract as in the Big 10, there has been considerably more red tape, given the various regulations and tuition differentials among the programs. These kinds of shared programs are desperately needed now, and the need for them can be expected to grow as the number of distance doctoral programs increases.

Delivering an online program differs in many ways from delivering a single course. It is necessary to create a program shell that not only allows branding of the program but also gives students a sense of place and access to the same support systems they would have if they were on campus. Because course management systems were designed to house individual courses, they do not always function as well to support an overall program. We had to add another layer over the actual course management system to support the program components. Although this layer is available in the course management system we purchased, other programs at The University of Arizona do not use it, which has made some functions more difficult for us, such as automatically populating students within courses.

The events of September 11, 2001 complicated online doctoral education for international students when visa restrictions became more stringent, requiring that students studying in this country, but enrolled in an online program, must take two face-to-face courses per semester. In addition, some countries still do not recognize online doctoral education.

Cultural differences among online students deserve more attention than they have received to date. Language and culture are closely linked, and online education is language intensive. International students may find the requirements for online discussion difficult because of language issues. In addition, these students must grapple with the different cultural connotations of terms. As a result, their level of interaction may be somewhat lower. On the other hand, asynchronous discussions benefit international students by allowing them time to check the meaning of terms, spelling, and grammar before posting responses. Dillon and colleagues[13] reported differences in learning styles partly attributable to culture. For example, in their study, students observed that Western students tend to be more actively involved than Eastern students. We have observed that international students sometimes struggle with critical evaluation because it is not commonly an expectation in education in some countries.

The cost of delivering online education is high because of the technology, technology support, student support, and course development. The relatively low number of students in a doctoral program as compared with undergraduate programs makes the cost per student even higher. Most distance doctoral programs impose an additional program or technology fee to recover some of the costs.

At The University of Arizona, we admit only full-time students, a decision made in large part to produce PhD graduates more quickly. Part-time study, in our experience, can go on for many years. Our students take at least nine credits per semester, with some additional course work during the summer. Although we urge students to cut back on work and other activities, and they are asked to describe how they intend to do so before their admission, many do not follow through and as a result they struggle to balance their education, work, and family commitments. Although most students manage to do this with amazing success, they pay a price educationally and personally (educationally by not allowing themselves time to explore more deeply or participate in research teams and personally by not having sufficient time to for rest and relaxation).

A growing number of schools are now offering the DNP degree at a distance in addition to, or instead of, a PhD. The competencies for this degree are just beginning to take shape, and the precise differences between the DNP and PhD continue to be debated. As a terminal clinical degree, however, the DNP requires clinical competencies that distinguish it from the PhD and are likely to require on-campus skill validation. Providing both degrees in the same program can strain schools' capacity to provide the number and kinds of options required by two differing programs. At The University of Arizona, we have engaged in several workshops to define and refine the PhD and DNP curricula, trying to discern which program outcomes are similar and which are unique to determine when we can pool faculty resources and when we cannot.

EVALUATION

Like others (eg,[14]), our faculty has found that online education provides advantages in expanding access to instructional resources, promoting active learning, increasing the pool of potential students, and increasing the level of participation in and the quality of class discussion. In part because we were given time to redesign courses, we found that redesigning our courses was a satisfying experience. On the other hand, we found that online teaching consumed more time, at least initially, and many of us felt that we were online all day long. Faculty and students alike sometimes missed the nonverbal cues of the classroom.

To date, there have been few evaluation studies of the online programs, in part because few programs have graduated sufficient students to measure outcomes. Halter and colleagues[15] used a phenomenologic approach and an interview methodology to explore the experience of five students enrolled in Malone College's online PhD program. Three themes were identified from the interview transcripts of five students:

> Considering the fit. Students reported basing some of their choices of programs on how the program fit with their other commitments (family, employment, and so forth). For many, moving to a face-to-face program was simply not an option. Other considerations were the learning environment; these students had carefully weighed whether they could learn effectively in an online environment.

Liking the fit. Respondents were positive about their experience, some noting that it fit their personalities because they were not pressured to respond quickly in a classroom but could be more reflective and intentional about their responses. In addition, some students felt that they were independent learners and did not need a lot of group support to succeed. One of the five reported feeling somewhat isolated at times, but felt that the convenience outweighed the isolation.

Making it fit. Respondents reported having to "learn new skills and modify old ones"[15] (p. 102) as they learned to use new technology and to communicate largely through text. The Malone program used a great deal of synchronous discussion (chat), and students found it difficult to type responses quickly without a lot of thinking, but learned to write succinctly and adopt abbreviations. (This result contrasts with our own experience, perhaps because we rely more on asynchronous discussion in which students have time to reflect on their responses before posting. Our faculty typically reports that student responses are of higher quality than they were in the classroom and that the responses come from all students, not just those who are more verbally confident.) Some of the students commented that there was nowhere to hide—everyone was expected to participate. Based on our own experience, this may be one of the real benefits of online discussions. Other respondents missed the nonverbal behaviors that would have been available in a face-to-face setting.

Although the study has limitations (eg, sample size, potential selection bias), the results are consistent (except as noted) with our experience. Overall, students in online doctoral programs have made conscious choices to obtain a doctorate by way of distance technology. Attrition has been low in our program, which suggests that students know their own learning capabilities and needs and that we have been able to meet those needs. Within our own program, we have encountered the range of life experiences: two births, an adoption, an unexpected student death, injuries, family issues, military call-ups, and so forth. Students and faculty have grown even closer as a result of sharing these experiences.

SUMMARY

Today several online programs are increasing nurses' access to doctoral education, both PhD and DNP. Initially distance doctoral programs were offered by private, non–research-intensive programs, but today online doctoral education is also offered by nursing programs at research-extensive universities. Nurses appreciate the convenience of these programs, and faculty members welcome the opportunity to work with a more diverse and talented cadre of students. Instructional and communication technologies exist to support teaching any subject effectively in an online setting, and to support research mentoring, although we have a great deal more experience in the former than in the latter. Our first student cohort is now completing the program. Along with others, we will be watching their careers closely as the ultimate measure of success.

REFERENCES

1. Leners DW, Wilson VW, Sitzman KL. Twenty-first century doctoral education: online with a focus on nursing education. Nurs Educ Perspect 2007;28(6):332–6.
2. National League for Nursing. Nursing data review, academic year 2005–2006: executive summary 2008. Available at: http://www.nln.org/research/datareview/executive_summary.pdf. Accessed March 7, 2008.

3. American Association of Colleges of Nursing (2007). Annual state of the schools. Available at: http://www.aacn.nche.edu/Media/pdf/AnnualReport07.pdf. Accessed February 29, 2008.
4. Edwardson S. Matching standards and needs in doctoral education in nursing. J Prof Nurs 2004;20(1):40–6.
5. Effken JA, Boyle JS, Isenberg MA. Creating a virtual research community: The University of Arizona PhD Program. To appear in: J Prof Nurs 2008, Jul–Aug.
6. Garrison DR, Anderson T, Archer W. Critical inquiry in a text-based environment: computer conferencing in higher education. The Internet and Higher Education 2000;2(2–3):87–105.
7. Rovai AP. Sense of community, perceived cognitive learning, and persistence in asynchronous learning networks. The Internet and Higher Education 2002;5(4): 319–32.
8. Thompson TL, MacDonald CJ. Community building, emergent design and expecting the unexpected: creating a quality eLearning experience. The Internet and Higher Education 2005;8(3):233–49.
9. Rovai AP. Development of an instrument to measure classroom community. The Internet and Higher Education 2002;5(3):197–211.
10. Shea P. A study of students' sense of learning community in online environments. Journal of Asynchronous Learning Networks 2006;10(10). Available at: http://www.sloan-c.org/publications/jaln/v10n1/v10n1_4shea_member.asp. Retrieved March 3, 2008.
11. Ivankova NV, Stick SL. Students' persistence in a distributed doctoral program in educational leadership in higher education: a mixed methods study. Research in Higher Education 2006;48(1):93–135.
12. Ice P, Curtis R, Phillips P, et al. Using asynchronous audio feedback to enhance teaching presence and students' sense of community. Journal of Asynchronous Learning Networks 2007;11(2):3–25.
13. Dillon P, Wang R, Tearle P. Cultural disconnection in virtual education. Pedagogy, Culture & Society 2007;15(2):153–74.
14. Cravener PA. Faculty experiences with providing online courses: thorns among the roses. Comput Nurs 1999;17(1):42–7.
15. Halter MJ, Kleiner C, Hess RF. The experience of nursing students in an online doctoral program in nursing: a phenomenological study. Int J Nurs Stud 2006; 43:99–105.

Transcultural Nursing Courses Online: Implications for Culturally Competent Care

Jamie E. Adam, MSN, RN, FNP, NP-C[a,b,*]

KEYWORDS

• Online courses • Transcultural • Cultural competence

Online education has gained attention and demand in recent years. It is not surprising that nursing programs would use this mode of learning to increase access to nursing education in a time of nursing shortage.[1] The National Advisory Council on Nurse Education and Practice estimates that by the year 2015, there will be 114,500 vacant, full-time registered nurse (RN) positions.[2] Fortunately, advances in technology and online education afford students the ability to pursue nursing courses with more ease and convenience, thereby encouraging enrollment into nursing programs. This may help target the working, adult student that comprises a growing portion of the undergraduate nursing student population.[3] This article explores the issues surrounding cultural diversity in nursing curriculum and the potential for online nursing curriculum to competently address these issues.

CHALLENGES OF DIVERSITY

To add to the challenge of diversity in nursing education, the American population is becoming increasingly diverse, while nurse ethnicity has diversified very little. The RN population in the United States is 90% White, with the remaining 10% Hispanic, Black, Asian/Pacific Islander, or Native American/Alaskan Native.[4,5] This creates much concern among experts for delivering culturally competent care. It has been suggested that this lack of minority representation among health professionals has contributed to the persistent health disparities seen in the United States.[6]

The National Advisory Council on Nurse Education and Practice offers that a major strategy to reduce disparities in America is to increase the number of minority nurses.[2]

[a] School of Nursing, Middle Tennessee State University, Murfreesboro, TN, USA
[b] Primary Care & Hope Clinic, Murfreesboro, TN, USA
* 258 Trinity Road, Branson, MO 65616.
E-mail address: jamieadam02@yahoo.com

Nurs Clin N Am 43 (2008) 567–574
doi:10.1016/j.cnur.2008.06.006
0029-6465/08/$ – see front matter © 2008 Elsevier Inc. All rights reserved.

This strategy seems compelling with the data that diverse populations seek health care providers that are of similar background and use appropriate health care services when diverse providers are present.[7] In addition, compliance rates and patient outcomes are better when providers are communicating in the patient's language.[8]

Although the health care industry needs a more diversified workforce, recruiting and retaining minority nursing students has proven to be difficult. In fact, attrition rates range from 15% to 85% among minority students. One nursing program in New Jersey went from 76 students to 26 students by the end of the first semester. In this particular case, the New Jersey school boasts a 90% to 100% National Council Licensure Examination (NCLEX) passing rate.[9] Pacquiao[9] argues that the Board of Nursing's primary focus is on the NCLEX passing rate with little attention to the attrition rate. Lack of faculty support, Eurocentric curriculum, and feeling of powerlessness are all possible factors in attrition rates.[10,11]

Subsequently, the lack of student diversity only adds to the problem of understanding cultural differences when there is very little cultural diversity in the learning environment.[12] A study by Etowa and colleagues[13] noted that nursing students are more likely to provide culturally competent care when having studied and practiced in a diverse nursing student population.

RESPONSE TO DIVERSITY CHALLENGES

There is no question that culturally competent care is needed, only how to best approach cultural care in nursing curriculum.[14] The American Nurses Association Council on Cultural Diversity in Nursing Practice, the Transcultural Nursing Society, and the Council on Nursing and Anthropology are three primary nursing organizations that have supported improving cultural competence, diversity in nursing, and cultural aspects in curriculum. In 1977, the National League for Nursing was one of the first funding and accrediting bodies to mandate cultural content within nursing curriculum.[15]

At present, both the National League for Nursing (NLN) and the American Association of Colleges of Nursing (AACN) require curricula in cultural competence in undergraduate and graduate nursing programs.[15] The Office of Minority Health within the US Department of Health & Human Services released the National Standards on Culturally and Linguistically Appropriate Services (CLAS). The 14 standards are divided into themes of organization supports, access services, and culturally competent care.[16] Recently the Joint Commission on Accreditation of Health care Organizations (JCAHO) included requirements to assess communication needs and the patient's primary language.[17]

TRANSCULTURAL CURRICULUM

In response to the need for cultural skills in a diverse health care population, most nursing programs have been incorporating cultural content throughout their curriculum. However, in many programs, only one or two faculty members are responsible for this integration. In addition, although several models for transcultural nursing exist, it is not known which models schools are using, if any.[18] As a result, there is wide variation among nursing programs in how cultural competence is incorporated. Some programs are able to offer courses specifically focused on transcultural nursing concepts. For programs such as these, there has been controversy about whether transcultural nursing can be taught in an online format (Campinha-Bacote, personal communication, 2007).

ADVANTAGES OF AN ONLINE COURSE

Online technologies have been and are still being used to supplement many traditional classroom courses. E-mail, Internet list-serves, World Wide Web, and video/audio conferencing are often used to supplement materials and learning activities.[3] A growing number of nursing programs are offering courses entirely online.[3] Online courses may give nursing programs an advantage in recruiting students, especially adult learners.[1,3] Student advantages include convenience, less travel time, and more time to balance school with work and family.[1] Online learning provides a non-threatening environment that encourages discussion, possibly even more so by students who would be quiet and reserved in traditional classrooms. Students also have the comfort of accessing online courses anywhere, anytime.[19]

Russell[20] reported that learning outcomes among traditional students versus distance learning students showed no significant differences. That being said, data suggest that many students and faculty prefer distance learning.[1,21] Zembylas and Vrasidas[22] note the testimony of a student gaining access to other cultural values via online communication with classmates separated by the Pacific Ocean. Without online capabilities, interactions such as these would not be possible.

In the case of implementing transcultural courses, the online format offers several advantages to nursing programs. Online courses provide the opportunity for institutions to collaborate and share expertise specific to their institution.[3] Students and faculty have the potential to represent diverse ethnic and cultural backgrounds. For example, Excelsior College offers an entirely "virtual" nursing program, composed of approximately 17,000 students from a variety of locations.[18] A virtual classroom affords students the ability to communicate not only from city to city but from another state or even country.

A major concern for transcultural nursing educators is whether communication and group interaction can effectively occur in an online format. Experts argue that this is possible. Discussion board formats allow students to expound on topics, allowing time for students to review their own comments, and revise unclear statements. A written record of the conversations allows students to reread comments later to better understand the meanings of postings.[19] Also, electronic communication provides a safe medium for students and faculty to confront each other.[21] Students gain a sense of being part of the group by seeing the responses of other students.[1] In addition, faculty members have the opportunity to provide feedback and acknowledge each student's comments equally.[22]

Kenny[19] conducted research on participant interaction within an online focus group. The purpose of the study was to identify if group interaction and active engagement could occur in an online format. The study involved 38 Australian nurses communicating via computer over an 8-week timeframe. The researcher posed discussion questions for participants, while participants responded to these questions and posted questions of their own. Findings of the study included active participation by all participants with most accessing the discussion site at least once a day and making a total of 263 postings. Participants commented that the experience was addictive and enjoyable. The researcher expressed this opportunity as a positive experience that yielded fruitful group interaction and individual participation.

CONCERNS WITH AN ONLINE COURSE

There are some notable challenges with online education. For a summary of advantages and disadvantages, see **Box 1**. Cost to the student and to the university is a concern. Although newer technologies are becoming more affordable, retiring existing technologies to acquire them is a great overall cost to the university. Another challenge to the university is federal financial aid regulations. Currently federal regulations will allow students to complete online courses with student federal financial aid. However

---

Box 1
Advantages and disadvantages to online curriculum

Advantages

Able to recruit more students

Appeal to adult learners

Convenient for many; may access the course anywhere, anytime

Less travel time

Nonthreatening environment

May encourage discussion from shy students

Students gain a sense of feeling part of a group

No significant difference in learning outcomes

Students able to gain exposure to classmates from another state, region, or country

May offer diverse faculty, shared expertise

Discussion board allows deeper understanding of comments and encourages individual feedback

Disadvantages

Increased cost to students

May require new technology and therefore may increase cost to institution

May conflict with federal financial aid regulations

Cannot monitor attendance as easily

Poor computer skills may provide a challenge to some students

Time zone differences among students and faculty may limit certain online formats

Requires student to navigate Web site for "hidden" information

May require more time for faculty to respond to students individually or to respond to questions, for example

Requires faculty to maintain and update Web site frequently

Plagiarism with online paper mills may be an issue

Online curriculum cannot fully replace face-to-face interaction

---

universities must not offer more than 50% of courses online or allow more than 50% of students to be enrolled in online classes at any one time. In addition, the institution must document attendance, which becomes difficult in an online course.[3] To help with financial aid for individual students, some programs have chosen to require computers, thus making it feasible to roll into a financial aid package.

Online education requires computer access and basic computer skills of the student. This can be a hindrance for some students.[19] Online education is available in synchronous (live) or asynchronous (fixed, preprepared) coursework modes.[23] Students that are less computer efficient may have difficulty keeping up with a live chat among several students. Also, time zone differences between student locations, especially with international students may pose a disadvantage to the synchronous format.

In addition, navigating course Web sites can be difficult for students not familiar to the Internet. Faculty have reported spending more time in an online course than in the traditional classroom because of numerous e-mails from students asking for clarification of course information, and so forth.[1] In addition, maintaining and updating Web sites that may become disabled during a course can be time consuming.[19] Another rising concern nursing faculty report is plagiarism by students using prewritten online paper mills. Fortunately, most faculty members have access to Web sites such as plagiarism.org and turnitin.com that will scan written assignments for plagiarism.[1] An online transcultural nursing course has some important limitations. Campinha-Bacote offers that a key part of becoming culturally competent involves actual, face-to-face cultural encounters (Campinha-Bacote, personal communication, 2007). The question has been posed, "Can students learn to relate well in a multidisciplinary environment when their dominant educational experiences have been technology-based, essentially isolated from classmates and teachers except for telecommunications?."[3] Regardless of the answer, it is unlikely that students will learn all that is necessary about transcultural nursing within the virtual classroom. It is important to note that a student is not an expert on a culture after being exposed to 3 or 4 members from another ethic group.[24] Therefore, a course environment, even diversified cannot substitute an actual cultural encounter.

Likewise, case study scenarios or simulations are generally lacking a holistic view of a patient's cultural background. Simulations may focus entirely on the nurse-patient encounter and miss the economic, social, and political contexts that surround the patients' abilities to obtain treatment or maintain their cultural beliefs.[18] In addition, some experts caution that students will specifically seek interactions that will earn them a good grade.[22] These "staged" online interactions may taint the spontaneity and honesty of group discussion.

TIPS FOR ONLINE COURSE SUCCESS

There are some general tips to having a successful online course. For students that have trouble navigating learning modules, faculty can provide additional "help" links to redirect students to the correct location.[21] Faculty can use synchronous chat times for classroom discussions and faculty office hours. Posting weekly tasks on an online discussion board can help clarify student expectations and avoid confusion.[1] Regular monitoring of Web links and course "upkeep" are factors in teaching online courses.[21] Faculty have an ethical responsibility to acknowledge student contributions without showing partiality.[22] Data suggest that a sense of connectedness is critical for online students.[25]

There are several tips from the experts to increase the success and effectiveness of an online transcultural nursing courses. Unanimously, experts agree that an experiential learning activity is key to developing cultural competence.[9,14,24,26,27] Students must have personal, hands-on experiences with different cultures; however, learning activities should be structured and precepted by faculty-appointed professionals. Student-directed activities allow for too much variability and a possibility of missing the objectives of the activity. Dr. Campinha-Bacote cautions that student-directed cultural experiences may leave too much room for interpretation. "A student might feel she has satisfied a Mexican cultural experience by attending a fiesta and eating a taco" (Campinha-Bacote, personal communication, 2007).

Dually noted, too much structure may limit the amount of opportunity the student has to practice culturally competent skills.[26] There are a variety of learning activities that would provide a balanced atmosphere for cultural learning. Activities may include assisting community agencies that serve diverse populations.[18] Community events such as health fairs and forums allow students to learn textbook cultural content firsthand.[26] Many nursing programs teach cultural competence by requiring students to have a cultural immersion experience. Some students commute daily to another community for a cultural experience.[18] Excelsior College has students submit a videotape of a teaching session with a culturally diverse group.[18] Students may display poster projects demonstrating cultural concepts in hospitals and community agencies.[12]

In addition to experiential learning, online modules or practice scenarios can help students integrate theory and practice.[28] The addition of audio to online lectures may also improve learning of cultural content. A randomized trial by Spickard and colleagues[29] evaluated the impact of online lecture with and without audio. The researchers measured the time, satisfaction, and knowledge of 3- and 4-year medical students watching online video lectures with and without audio. The findings of the trial demonstrated that students with the audio feed took longer to complete the lecture but reported greater satisfaction with the lecture experience, and showed higher knowledge scores.

Other helpful tools for nursing institutions and faculty include consulting the AACN White Paper regarding distance technology in nursing education. The AACN published guidelines regarding planning, faculty development, student support, technology infrastructure, and evaluation of outcomes concerning online courses in nursing education. The guidelines pose questions for administrators to address before setting up a distance technology program.[3] In addition to consulting the guidelines, faculty members should have preparation and continuing education in cultural content.[18] Schools should seek to diversify faculty and encourage international assignments for faculty and students.[30] **Table 1** lists further resources and Web sites on cultural competence.

FUTURE IMPLICATIONS

Teaching and learning cultural competence is a moral obligation. To eliminate health disparities, we must begin with educational institutions.[31] "Change at the school level creates the next generation of practitioners for whom cultural care is not the exception or reverse discrimination, but is the norm."[14] We can assume that the degree of a student's cultural competence is related to the type and amount of exposure to other culture groups.[27] As faculty we need to provide cultural opportunities for our students to gain cultural skills. Chrisman[14] suggests a holistic approach to cultural competence. He argues that cultural competence is easier to sustain with partnerships among educational institutions, health care agencies, and the community. Programs

Table 1 Cultural competence resources and web sites	
Organization	**Web Site**
Center for Cross-Cultural Health	http://www.crosshealth.com
Culturedmed	http://www.sunyit.edu/library/html/culturedmed/
Diversity Rx	http://www.DiversityRx.org/
Cossmho Hispanic Health Link	http://www.hispanichealth.org/
Cross Cultural Health Care Program	http://xculture.org/
The Black Health Network	http://www.blackhealthnetwork.com/
Transcultural and Multicultural Health Links	http://www.lib.iun.indiana.edu/trannurs.htm
Transcultural Nursing	http://www.culturediversity.org
Native Web	http://www.nativeculture.com
Ethnomed	http://www.healthlinks.washington.edu/clinical/ethnomed
Office of Minority Health. U.S. Dept of HHS	http://www.omhrc.gov

targeting K–12 are necessary to attract diverse students to the health care workforce and will require a unified effort to be effective.[7,9] Although several qualitative studies have demonstrated increased patient satisfaction with culturally competent care, research is strongly needed in demonstrating further consequences of cultural competence in schools and the workforce.[14]

SUMMARY

Today's advances and opportunities in technology provide an excellent opportunity for nursing programs in the United States to incorporate online courses as a means of meeting the demands of culturally competent curriculum. With little diversity in the workforce or nursing student population, students need opportunities to learn essential cultural competence skills to care for an increasingly diverse patient population. Online transcultural nursing courses offer an avenue for students to acquire these skills. By using effective online teaching techniques, faculty can provide their students with a transcultural nursing course experience that will prepare them to provide culturally competent care.

REFERENCES

1. Moore P, Hart L. Strategies for teaching nursing research online. International council of nurses. Int Nurs Rev 2004;51:123–8.
2. American Association of Colleges of Nursing. AACN white paper: distance technology in nursing education. 2005. Available at: http://aacn.nche.edu/Publications/positions/whitepaper.htm. Accessed June 18, 2007.
3. American Nurses Association. Ethics and human rights position statements: discrimination an racism in health care. 1998. Available at: http://nursingworld.org/readroom/position/ethics/prtcldv.htm. Accessed June 18, 2007.
4. U.S. Census Bureau. The white population: 2000. Available at: http://www.census.gov/prod/2001pubs/c2kbr01-4.pdf. Accessed June 18, 2007.
5. Sullivan LW. Missing persons: minorities in the health professions. A report of the The Sullivan Commission on diversity in the healthcare workforce 2004. Available at: http://admissions.duhs.duke.edu/sullivancommission/index.htm. Accessed August 10, 2007.
6. National Advisory Council on Nurse Education and Practice. A national agenda for nursing workforce racial/ethnic diversity; 2000. Washington, DC. U.S. Department of Health and Human Services, Bureau of Health Professions.
7. Gilchrist KL, Rector C. Can you keep them? Strategies to attract and retain nursing students from diverse populations: best practices in nursing education. J Transcult Nurs 2007;18(3):277–85.
8. Simpson RL. Recruit, retain, assess: technology's role in diversity. Nurs Adm Q 2004;28(5):217–20.
9. Pacquiao D. The relationship between cultural competence education and increasing diversity in nursing schools and practice settings. J Transcult Nurs 2007;18(1):28S–37S.
10. Yoder M. Instructional responses to ethnically diverse nursing students. J Nurs Educ 1996;35(7):315–21.
11. Davidhizar R, Dowd SB, Giger JN. Educating the culturally diverse healthcare student. Nurse Educ 1998;23(20):38–42.
12. Hughes KH, Hood LJ. Teaching methods and an outcome tool for measuring cultural sensitivity in undergraduate nursing students. J Transcult Nurs 2007;18(1):57–62.

13. Etowa JB, Foster S, Vukic AR, et al. Recruitment and retention of minority students: diversity in nursing education. Int J Nurs Educ Scholarsh 2005. Available at: http://www.bepress.com/ijnes/vol2/iss1/art13. Accessed June 18, 2007.
14. Chrisman NJ. Extending cultural competence through systems change: academic, hospital, and community partnerships. J Transcult Nurs 2007;18(1): 68S–76S.
15. DeSantis LA, Lipson JG. Brief history of inclusion of content on culture in nursing education. J Transcult Nurs 2007;18(1):7S–9S.
16. Office of Minority Health. National standards on culturally and linguistically appropriate services (CLAS); n.d. Washington, DC. U.S. Department of Health and Human Services.
17. Joint Commission Resources. Comprehensive accreditation manual for hospitals: the official handbook. Table of changes. 2007. Available at: http://www.jcrinc. com/26813/newsletters/28192/. Accessed June 18, 2007.
18. Lipson JG, Desantis LA. Current approaches to integrating elements of cultural competence in nursing education. J Transcult Nurs 2007;18(1):10S–20S.
19. Kenny AJ. Methodological issues in nursing research. Interaction in cyberspace: an online focus group. J Adv Nurs 2005;49(4):414–22.
20. Russell TL. The no significant difference phenomenon. Raleigh (NC): North Carolina State University 1999.
21. Huckstadt A, Hayes K. Evaluation of interactive online courses for advanced practice nurses. J Am Acad Nurse Pract 2005;17(3):85–9.
22. Zembylas M, Vrasidas C. Levinas and the "inter-face": the ethical challenge of online education. Educ Theory 2005;55(1):61–78.
23. American Association of Colleges of Nursing. AACN Issue Bulletin. Distance learning is changing and challenging nursing education 2000. Available at: http://www.aacn.nche.edu/Publications/issues/jan2000.htm. Accessed June 18, 2007.
24. Campinha-Bacote J. Many faces: addressing diversity in healthcare. Online J Issues Nurs 2003. Available at: http://www.nursingworld.org/ojin/topic20/ tpc20_2.htm. Accessed June 18, 2007.
25. Shin N, Chan J. Direct and indirect effects of online learning on distance education. Br J Educ Technol 2004;35(3):275–88.
26. Anderson NL, Calvillo ER, Fongwa MN. Community-based approaches to strengthen cultural competency in nursing education and practice. J Transcult Nurs 2007;18(1):49S–59S.
27. Schim SM, Doorenbos A, Benkert R, et al. Culturally congruent care: putting the puzzle together. J Transcult Nurs 2007;18(2):103–10.
28. Dyson S. Transcultural health care practice: core practice module, chapter three: transcultural nursing care of adults. Royal College of Nursing. n.d. Available at: http://www.rcn.org/uk/resources/transcultural/adulthealth/index.php. Accessed June 18, 2007.
29. Spickard A, Smithers J, Cordray D, et al. A randomized trial of an online lecture with and without audio. Med Educ 2004;38:787–90.
30. De Leon Siantz ML, Meleis AI. Integrating cultural competence into nursing education and practice: 21st century action steps. J Transcult Nurs 2007;18(1): 86S–90S.
31. Giger J, Davidhizar RE, Purnell L, et al. American Academy of Nursing expert panel report: developing cultural competence to eliminate health disparities in ethnic minorities and other vulnerable populations. J Transcult Nurs 2007;18(2): 95–102.

Visual Literacy in the Online Environment

Sandra J. Mixer, PhD, RN[a],*, Marilyn R. McFarland, PhD, RN, FNP-BC, CTN[b],
Leigh Ann McInnis, PhD, FNP-BC[c]

KEYWORDS

• Visual literacy • Nursing education • Online education

Although nurse educators are experts in their area of specialty and in the discipline of nursing, many do not understand how to apply the principles of visual literacy to effectively teach. Nurses and nurse educators receive information regarding verbal communication but little or no education regarding visual communication or visual literacy. Visual literacy can be used by nurse educators to enhance learner perception and support learner cognition.[1] In today's learning environment, students are technologically savvy and visual stimulation is an expectation.

This article describes the use of visual literacy as a tool to enhance student learning. Concepts that provide a framework for understanding visual literacy, including repetition, integration, hierarchy, and simplicity, are described. The effectiveness of visual literacy is also discussed, followed by a presentation of a visual literacy tool created to teach transcultural nursing and the culture care theory to nursing students in an online environment. A review of the challenges encountered, use and critique of the tool by nurse educators across the country, and a process for continuing evaluation conclude the article. A copy of the visual literacy teaching tool is made available to readers using the URL address on the World Wide Web.

The Internet became available to most individuals less than a decade ago. It has greatly changed the learning experience of a typical nursing student. Today's student uses laptops, instant messaging, blogs, and cell phones to find information and to stay connected. Rapid changes in technology and health care intersect for our students, creating a dynamic learning environment. This environment necessitates a change in the way we, as educators, approach teaching and learning.

In the past, a successful student mastered reading, writing, mathematics, and basic nursing knowledge. In today's world, static knowledge is obsolete. Lifelong learning is

[a] College of Nursing, University of Tennessee, 120 Volunteer Boulevard, Knoxville, TN 37996, USA
[b] School of Nursing, University of Michigan, Flint, MI, 2180 William S. White Building, Flint, MI 48502, USA
[c] School of Nursing, Middle Tennessee State University, 1500 Greenland Drive, Box 81, Murfreesboro, TN 37132, USA
* Corresponding author.
E-mail address: ksmixer@yahoo.com (S.J. Mixer).

Nurs Clin N Am 43 (2008) 575–582
doi:10.1016/j.cnur.2008.06.010   nursing.theclinics.com
0029-6465/08/$ – see front matter © 2008 Elsevier Inc. All rights reserved.

now the expectation for all individuals. The technologies of today require a different skill set. Digital age literacy requires basic literacy (the three Rs), scientific literacy, economic literacy, technological literacy, visual literacy, information literacy, multicultural literacy, and global awareness.[2] All of these domains are components to successful lifelong learning. For students of today, visual images are just one of the numerous formats synonymous with technology.[3] The Net generation does not actually use technology—it is just an integral part of their lives. They expect visual stimulation in education.[4] In reality, simple visuals improve learning for most students. One should not take for granted, however, that a preference for visual entertainment is necessarily accompanied by superior understanding of visual information.[5,6] Although most individuals understand and learn from simple visuals, prior knowledge of concepts is required for complex visuals to be effective. Visual literacy beyond the printed text or discussion boards is thus particularly important in the context of teaching in the online environment.[2,7,8]

VISUAL LITERACY

Visual literacy is a complex phenomenon. Although individuals may conceptualize visual literacy as visual images, in reality visual literacy combines words and graphics to enhance learning. Visual literacy is "the ability to understand and use images, including the ability to think, learn, and express oneself in terms of images".[1] Visual literacy involves designing visuals to enhance learner perception and support learner cognition. Visuals improve communication of ideas.[9–11] Examples of the use of visual literacy in nursing education are PowerPoint slides, film clips, handouts, animations, symbols, posters, streaming video, DVDs, web pages, and syllabi. These examples may use combinations of words, images, and audio.

Research shows that most individuals can remember images better than words and the combination of images and words enhances learning.[1] Visuals are effective in learning because they facilitate memory processes and assist students in organizing information in a way they can remember.[11] Graphics and visual images help visual learners comprehend otherwise complex concepts. People learn from simple visuals. Complex visuals are effective when the learner has some prior knowledge about the concepts. Visual images are particularly effective for improving learning when addressing the needs of individuals who have visual-spatial cognitive learning styles.[5,11] As we consider the elements of visual literacy, it is essential to incorporate a balance between visual and verbal cues when using new technologies.[11]

There are many components of visual literacy. Several key concepts that provide a framework for understanding visual literacy are repetition, similarity, integration, hierarchy, and figure/ground. The principle of repetition entails using an element of a visual more than once in an effort to create harmony and unity. The principle of similarity refers to the mind's tendency to group things together based on likeness. Using the principles of repetition and similarity, a PowerPoint presentation would display the same background, colors, and shapes for each slide to create consistency and reduce cognitive load. This consistency allows the learner to focus on the content of the slide rather than spending time and energy being distracted by adjusting to a new screen each time.[9,12]

The principle of integration uses a combination of verbal and visual presentation to facilitate cognition.[1,9] Hierarchy involves organizing information in a way that allows the mind to "chunk" concepts, thus facilitating memory. Information may be placed in ranking or ladder formats to demonstrate the relationships among data. The use of arrows, outlines, or concept maps further demonstrates order of importance. The notion of figure/ground is used to emphasize content, to make it more noticeable. Important content in the image stands out through techniques such as contrast. Contrast and similar methods relieve the brain of having to organize information and facilitate storage/memory.[1,12]

Nurse educators generally think about searching for words on the World Wide Web using search engines, such as Google, AltaVista, or ask. One can search using the image feature and quickly find images related to a pertinent topic (L. Lohr, personal communication, 2007). Librarians provide an important resource for faculty, as they are experts in locating visual resources to magnify critical content.[13] These are simple ways to incorporate visual literacy. Visual literacy can take many forms. Following is an example of using visual literacy to teach transcultural nursing in an online environment.

VISUAL LITERACY EXAMPLE

An online educational technology course, taught by Lohr,[1] was taken by one of the authors and provided the impetus and inspiration to create a visual literacy tool to teach transcultural nursing and the culture care theory in an online environment. The goal of this project was to create visuals that would facilitate nursing students' and nurses' understanding of the culture care theory as depicted in the Sunrise Enabler. The culture care theory is a nursing theory useful for nurses in practice, education, administration, and research in a multicultural world where people want their cultural values and lifeways (the way a person lives daily life) understood. The theory and Sunrise Enabler guide nurses in assessment and actions and decisions (interventions) to provide culturally congruent care.[14] The Sunrise Enabler is a copyrighted graphic developed by Leininger to depict an integrated holistic view of the influencing dimensions and major concepts of her culture care theory (**Fig. 1**). It is a cognitive map to assist nurses in comprehending the theory.

The Sunrise Enabler visual was adapted using pictures to enhance learner perception and support learner cognition. Images were created as a teaching strategy to focus students on dimensions of the theory using graphics. The pictures incorporated into the Sunrise Enabler were developed to represent words and concepts that students, especially novice students, have found challenging. For example, the concepts of worldview, cultural and social structure dimensions (eg, use of technology and religious and philosophical values and beliefs), and daily lifeways were represented using pictures relating to learners' previous knowledge.[14] Drawing from previous experience helps learners make connections to new material, thereby improving learning.[1] For example, an eye with a world in it portrays worldview (**Fig. 2**). Worldview refers to the way in which people look out at the world or the lens they use to see their world.[14]

As the visuals were developed and tested with colleagues and students, it became clear that an introductory reading assignment or a lecture to go with the slides would be necessary for student comprehension. A decision was made to use Leininger's Sunrise Enabler and integrate the visual images using the combination of words and symbols to further reinforce learners' understanding and recall. Streaming video of a presentation about these concepts was added to provide further understanding and meaning. Verbal dialog between the instructors and students present during the audio-videotaping presentation provided additional clarification of concepts and examples of application to various clinical settings. This technique represents the principle of integration: combination of verbal and visual presentation to facilitate cognition.

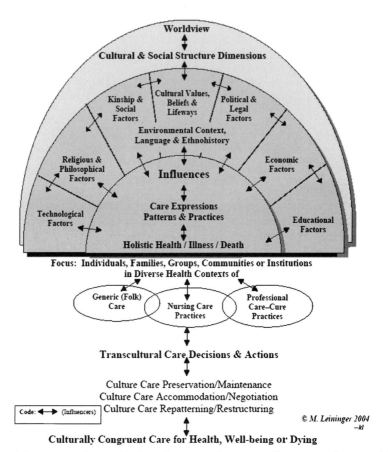

Fig. 1. Leininger's Sunrise Enabler to discover culture care. (*Courtesy of* Dr. Madeleine Leininger, Livonia, MI; with permission.)

This project combined streaming video (visual action and sound), PowerPoint slides (words and images), and graphics, which were used to teach transcultural nursing. The student could then proceed at his or her own pace, or use set timing. Learners can gain repeated exposure to the material based on their individual learning needs.[15] This teaching tool was intentionally created to be less than 20 minutes in length to maximize and hold the interest of students. This tool has been effectively used in

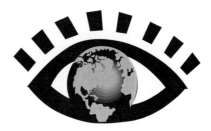

Fig. 2. Worldview.

online and in on-ground courses as a supplement to traditional face-to-face instruction in transcultural nursing and the culture care theory by faculty throughout the country. The tool can be embedded in a Web-based course platform using a URL link or CD. Readers may access this tool through the following Web site: http://www6.svsu.edu/~drr/tcn/producer_files/Default.htm. The authors request that if you choose to use the tool in your course, you would critique its usefulness and provide suggestions for refinement by sending a notice to ksmixer@yahoo.com.

As visuals for the Sunrise Enabler were developed, several challenges surfaced. Some phenomena were found to be too complex to be represented only by a visual (eg, culturally congruent care). Lohr[1] agrees that the importance of using words with images cannot be understated. Words may be the most efficient and effective way of communicating some concepts. Other challenges centered on creating visuals free of ethnocentrism. The challenge is using visuals worldwide because signs, symbols, and icons are not universally understood by all cultures. Research conducted in the United States found that clip art used in business presentations was often misunderstood, with cultural differences accounting for much of the variation in a symbol's meaning.[1]

VISUAL LITERACY AS A WORK IN PROGRESS

Visuals are always a work in progress. Using a model such as ACE (analyze, create, and evaluate) is essential in creating visuals that are relevant, meaningful, and effective.[1] The educator begins with analyzing the need for the visual. What does one want to communicate or teach? What context should be used? Does the learner have prior knowledge or is this new material? What is the purpose of this visual? Analysis may include a needs assessment or determining learner characteristics. The create step involves actually creating the visual: simple or complex, colors, text, image only, or combination. The educator may need to write text and find or create a graphic. The educator makes decisions about what to emphasize and how to organize information, and works to inspire the learner. Evaluation includes testing and editing. Feedback is solicited from experts and the intended audience/learners. The educator seeks to elicit how effective and appealing the visual is. Does the visual focus on the point or are there extraneous data to weed out?

The educator continues cycling through these steps (analyze, create, evaluate) until the visual is useful for teaching. Much like the steps in the nursing process, this process is nonlinear and multidimensional. Revision may continue to occur over time as the visual is used with numerous learners. As the evaluation process proceeds, "learning to let go"[1] is an important skill to use. Some visuals that are developed are not useful and need to be eliminated. As nurse educators, we see the struggle to let go in enormous PowerPoints that overwhelm students and confuse what the essential points are.

In the visual literacy example described for transcultural nursing, evaluation was solicited from numerous sources, representing hours of brainstorming. Critique was provided by Dr. Lohr, doctoral colleagues, transcultural nursing experts, nursing faculty and students, educational technology experts, the public, and Dr. Leininger (creator of the culture care theory and Sunrise Enabler). Principles of visual literacy were addressed. Because the Sunrise Enabler expresses numerous concepts, Dr. Lohr suggested brightening the portion of the image being expressed with graphics and dulling (fading), the remaining parts. Students provided feedback that this allowed them to follow the interplay of words and symbols. This observation emphasizes the importance of hierarchy (organizing information in order of importance) and figure/ground (making content noticeable).

These visuals were tested with senior nursing students in a leadership course and with registered nurse to bachelor of science in nursing and master of science in nursing students in a transcultural nursing course who were familiar with the culture care theory and Sunrise Enabler. Students provided feedback that the use of yellow was appropriate as it reflected the sunrise theme. They suggested that the white background was too harsh and should be light blue, which is softer and could symbolically represent the sky behind the sunrise. Second, they appreciated each section of the Sunrise Enabler being presented step-by-step and alternating between the Sunrise Enabler with words and visuals. Feedback from first-semester nursing students and pre-nursing students (who had no real knowledge of theory) was also solicited. Students liked the ease of being able to scan back and forth over the material to review sections by using the menu bar at the left of the presentation screen and the forward and backward arrows. Research results indicated that students using self-paced modules completed their work more quickly and were found to perform better than those using structured timed designs.[11] Active learning, self-direction, and multiple learning strategies are recommended in online education.[15]

In her evaluation, Dr. Madeline Leininger shared that the world in the eye symbol for worldview clarified this concept. She concurred with our challenges and suggested we continue to work to find more universal images. Additionally, Dr. Leininger was concerned about presenting the Sunrise Enabler broken down into steps because students might miss the gestalt of the enabler. In general, she shared that using pictures was an innovative idea to teach the culture care theory.

We continue to address the challenge of how to universally represent holistic health, dying, and culturally congruent care. Feedback from a doctoral colleague included a comment that the slide used to represent these three concepts was powerful. This feedback addresses the principles of content and working to communicate the essence of the theoretic concepts through images.

Using the ACE process, this visual literacy tool can be further improved. The streaming video quality is amateurish. A standard video recorder was used and neither the faculty presenters nor the student participants used a microphone, which resulted in limited sound quality and therefore affected the quality of the visual literacy explanation.

SUMMARY

Research supports the effectiveness of using visual literacy. The Sunrise Enabler example provides an opportunity to demonstrate the effectiveness of using visual literacy to teach in an online environment. Because students are immersed in digital literacy and multimodal learning, it is time for educators to embrace visual literacy. We must strike out beyond printed text, PowerPoint slides, and discussion boards to engage our students.

ACKNOWLEDGMENTS

This project was only possible based on the collaboration and synergy of many. Dr. Madeline Leininger is the founder of transcultural nursing and creator of the culture care theory and Sunrise Enabler. Dr. Linda Lohr was the teacher and author of *Creating Graphics for Learning and Performance*: *Lessons in Visual Literacy*, whose educational technology course provided the inspiration and opportunity for this project. Deborah Roberts is a masters-prepared instructional technology specialist who provided the technical expertise for this project, and Kristine Roethlisberger, RN, MSN, volunteered her time to be the videographer.

REFERENCES

1. Lohr LL. Creating graphics for learning and performance. Upper Saddle River (NJ): Pearson Education; 2003.
2. McDougal J. Engaging the visual generation: some Queensland teachers come to terms with changing literacies. Screen Education 2007;46:130–7. Available at: http://0-web.ebscohost.com.source.unco.edu/ehost/pdf?vid=5&hid=7&sid= d633870d-8ba1-4f09-9c53-08fb23d97514%40sessionmgr8. Accessed October 16, 2007.
3. Northcut KM. The relevance of Feenberg's critical theory of technology to critical visual literacy: the case of scientific and technical illustrations. J Tech Writ Comm [serial online] 2007;37(3):253–66. Available at: http://0-web.ebscohost.com.source.unco.edu/ehost/pdf?vid=6&hid=7&sid=d633870d-8ba1-4f09-9c53-08fb23d97514%40 sessionmgr8. Accessed October 14, 2007.
4. Maier CD, Kampf C, Kastberg P. Multimodal analysis: an integrative approach for scientific visualizing on the web. J Tech Writ Comm [serial online] 2007;37(4):453–78. Available at: http://0-web.ebscohost.com.source.unco.edu/ehost/pdf?vid=21& hid=7&sid=d633870d-8ba1-4f09-9c53-08fb23d97514%40sessionmgr8. Accessed October 16, 2007.
5. Messaris P. New literacies in action: visual education. Read Online 2001;4(7). Available at: http://www.readingonline.org/newliteracies/lit_index.asp?HREF=/ newliteracies/action/messaris/index.html. Accessed October 28, 2007.
6. Messaris P. Visual literacy in cross-cultural perspective. In: Kubey R, editor. Media literacy in the information age. Transaction Publishers 1996:135–62. Available at: Communication & Mass Media Complete, Ipswich, MA. Accessed October 28, 2007.
7. Bonk CJ, Zhang K. Introducing the R2D2 model: online learning for the diverse learners of this world. Dist Educ [serial online] 2006;27(2):249–64. Available at: http://0-web.ebscohost.com.source.unco.edu/ehost/pdf?vid=11&hid=7&sid= d633870d-8ba1-4f09-9c53-08fb23d97514%40sessionmgr8. Accessed October 16, 2007.
8. Whitson BA, Hoang CD, Jie T, et al. Association for academic surgery: technology-enhanced interactive surgical education. J Surg Res [serial online] 2006;136(1):13–8. Available at: http://0-www.sciencedirect.com.source.unco.edu/science?_ob= ArticleURL&_udi=B6WM6-4M0BHV5-1&_user=2570487&_coverDate=11%2F30% 2F2006&_rdoc=1&_fmt=&_orig=search&_sort=d&view=c&_acct=C000057861 &_version=1&_urlVersion=0&_userid=2570487&md5=46f74b01769b6ea69afe754 3876fdd9d. Accessed October 10, 2007.
9. Dunsworth Q, Atkinson RK. Fostering mulitmedia learning of science: exploring the role of an animated agent's image. Comput Educ [serial online] 2007;49(3):677–90. Available at: http://0-www.sciencedirect.com.source.unco.edu/science?_ob= ArticleURL&_udi=B6VCJ-4HWX8PY-2&_user=2570487&_coverDate=11%2F30% 2F2007&_rdoc=1&_fmt=&_orig=search&_sort=d&view=c&_acct=C000057861 &_version=1&_urlVersion=0&_userid=2570487&md5=5157721e2bcab4f942c326 6df7d7e188. Accessed October 14, 2007.
10. McCrudden M, Schraw G, Lehman S, et al. The effect of causal diagrams on text learning. Contemp Educ Psychol [serial online] 2007;32(3):367–88. Available at: http://0-www.sciencedirect.com.source.unco.edu/science?_ob=ArticleURL&_udi= B6WD1-4J32JB1-1&_user=2570487&_coverDate=07%2F31%2F2007&_rdoc= 1&_fmt=&_orig=search&_sort=d&view=c&_acct=C000057861&_version= 1&_urlVersion=0&_userid=2570487&md5=185619e61ce04d34847ab57d699e209b. Accessed October 12, 2007.

11. Stokes S. Visual literacy in teaching and learning: a literature perspective. Electron J Integrat Tech Educ 2002;1(1):10–9. Available at: http://ejite.isu.edu/ Volume1No1/Stokes.html. Accessed October 28, 2007.

12. Kinchin I. Developing PowerPoint handouts to support meaningful learning. Br J Educ Technol [serial online] 2006;37(4):647–50. Available at: http://0-web.ebscohost.com. source.unco.edu/ehost/pdf?vid=23&hid=7&sid=d633870d-8ba1-4f09-9c53-08fb23d97514%40sessionmgr8. Accessed October 14, 2007.

13. Davis-Kahl S, Banks KH. Analyzing the dynamics of race with information & visual literacy: a virtual poster session for Eye to I: visual literacy meets information literacy. 2007. Available at: http://www.iwu.edu/~sdaviska/ala2007/analyzingdynamics. html. Accessed October 28, 2007.

14. Leininger MM. Culture care diversity and universality theory and evolution of the ethnonursing method. In: Leininger MM, McFarland MR, editors. Culture care diversity & universality: a worldwide nursing theory. 2nd edition. New York: Jones and Bartlett; 2006. p. 1–41.

15. Jairath N, Mills ME. Online health science education: development & implementation. Philadelphia: Lippincott Williams & Wilkins; 2006.

Back to the Future: Personal Digital Assistants in Nursing Education

Renee P. McLeod, DNSc, APRN, BC, CPNP*, Mary Z. Mays, PhD

KEYWORDS

- Personal digital assistant • Mobile decision support
- Mobile technology • Handheld computing

Personal digital assistants (PDAs) have been a part of health care since they came on the market in the 1980s as an organizing device that could be carried easily in a pocket.[1–6] Today "PDA" represents a large number of hardware devices that range from a simple organizer to interactive wireless devices with two-way communication. These devices include an entire range of smartphones from companies such as Palm, Hewlett-Packard, LG, Nokia, Sony, Research in Motion (RIM), and Apple. Today's PDAs have the ability to download software, store files, record voice, play music and videos, and access the Internet; in short, they have most of the functions of a laptop computer. Unlike desktop or laptop computers they are small enough to fit easily into a pocket and are instant-on, instant-access devices.

Newer PDAs (eg, iPhone, Treo, Palm T/X, HP iPAQ) access the Internet to download files, retrieve information, and update software programs directly on the device without having to connect to a desktop or laptop computer. The Blackberry from RIM revised thinking in the marketplace by creating "push e-mail" for the PDA. The most recent handheld device, the Amazon Kindle, is marketed as an electronic reader with a slightly larger form factor than a typical PDA. The Kindle is an informatics warehouse that provides free access to the Internet, downloads e-books, articles, and blogs, searches them, and allows the reader to make notes on them. Newspapers, blogs, and magazines are pushed to the device. The Kindle is the first device to bridge

Financial disclosure: Dr. McLeod has consulted or been sponsored at presentations in the past by Palm, Lexi-Comp, and Skyscape. She currently has no direct financial interest in companies or products discussed in the article or in a competing company or product. Dr. Mays has no direct financial interest in companies or products discussed in the article or in a competing company or product.
Office of Transformational Technologies and Organizations, College of Nursing & Healthcare Innovation, Arizona State University, Mail Code 3020, 500 North 3rd Street, Phoenix, AZ 85004, USA
* Corresponding author.
E-mail address: renee.mcleod@asu.edu (R.P. McLeod).

Nurs Clin N Am 43 (2008) 583–592
doi:10.1016/j.cnur.2008.06.008
0029-6465/08/$ – see front matter © 2008 Elsevier Inc. All rights reserved.
nursing.theclinics.com

the gap between PDA and computer to change the way people access and read materials in a digital world.

The challenge for nursing education is to harness the power of PDAs to empower students to navigate, evaluate, select, and synthesize information to support real-time evidenced-based practice at the point of care. A secondary challenge is to be able to provide adequate support for students and faculty so that PDA use becomes a positive experience.

HISTORY OF PERSONAL DIGITAL ASSISTANTS IN HEALTH CARE

The current cycle of PDA evolution is illustrated in **Fig. 1**. Nurses, like the general population, first used PDAs as time management tools (#1 in **Fig. 1**) (ie, as personal organizers that were lighter and more efficient than paper and pencil notebooks).[7–14] Although Psion and Apple had early entries into the market, devices using the Palm operating system were the first devices to be used widely by clinicians in practice.[1,2] PDAs allowed clinicians to combine their flash cards, cheat sheets, notebooks, and schedulers into a single digital space that could be taken everywhere (#2 in **Fig. 1**). Early adopters saw the potential to move from having a pager, index cards, and cell phone in their pockets to carrying only one device—one with the potential to support finding answers to complex clinical questions at the point of care.[2,5,7,8,14] The power to create and record clinical pearls on the spot ensured that the devices would remain on the scene, but the ability to share information immediately by beaming information from one PDA to another cemented their place in the health care system.

Improvements in screens, battery life, and memory led to the production of reference books for the PDA, a simple export from book to e-book, a more mobile form factor.[8] With the development of true database applications suitable for the PDA, a few innovators realized the potential of PDAs to automate clinical tasks at the point of care. The group of enterprise solutions that emerged from these early attempts to make clinicians more mobile and efficient ensured the commercial viability of PDAs in health care.[13,15–19] The true tipping point in the evolution of PDAs, however, was the provision of ubiquitous wireless Internet connectivity and the consequent development of mobile browsers that enabled users to access online databases of clinical logs, health records, evidence-based guidelines, and peer-reviewed journals. These applications can be leveraged to support real-time, evidenced-based practice at the point of care.

Once PDAs were introduced into clinical practice, it became important to introduce the technology into the classroom (#3 in **Fig. 1**) so that graduates could be integrated into clinical practice easily.[9,12,18,20–31] At the time that students were being introduced

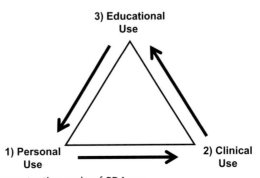

Fig. 1. Current self-perpetuating cycle of PDA use.

to PDAs in class, secular trends in cell phone technology and intensive smartphone marketing were ensuring a growing awareness of the devices by students. They were able to adopt them for personal use as time, contact, and digital music management tools.[7] This cycle from personal use to clinical use to educational use became self-perpetuating as the devices continued to evolve. Most nursing students today enter the program owning and using one or more of these devices, typically an Internet-enabled smartphone or digital music player.[2,7,9]

LITERATURE SEARCH STRATEGY

A literature search was conducted to identify the type of published information available on the use of PDAs in nursing education. Search strategies were focused on retrieving articles that specifically addressed measuring the impact of PDAs in nursing education. The final strategy (shown in **Box 1**) was used to search the Cumulative Index to the Nursing and Allied Health Literature (CINAHL) and the Medical Literature Analysis and Retrieval System Online (MEDLINE) databases.

The search of CINAHL yielded 69 articles and the search of MEDLINE yielded 67. Removal of duplicates within and across the two lists yielded 99 articles. Another 26 articles were discarded as irrelevant (eg, PDA referred to patent ductus arteriosus, pressurized direct aerosol, or participation in decision activities; handheld referred to diagnostic tool or patient's video game; technology studied was laptop, not PDA; study was on occupational safety of handheld devices; article was infomercial). The remaining 73 articles were used to identify the strength of the evidence for the use of PDAs in nursing education. Review of the articles revealed that half of them were single case-based discussions of how PDAs were implemented in nursing curricula (eg,[12,15,23,28–32]), a quarter were quasi-experimental tests of PDA functionality (eg,[7,9,16,24,33,34]), and a quarter were quasi-experimental tests of learning or patient outcomes (eg,[19,25,35–47]). No large-scale, randomized controlled tests of the PDA's efficacy in promoting positive changes in learning outcomes or novel changes in instructional practices were identified. A systematic review of the literature on the use of PDAs in medical education found a similar range of information.[48]

USING PERSONAL DIGITAL ASSISTANTS IN NURSING CURRICULA
Lessons Learned about Initial Implementation

The simplest way to initiate PDAs into a program is to require their use in a single course and to ask students to purchase the hardware of their choice and load a list

---

Box 1
Search strategy

Ovid CINAHL 1982 to Week 4 March 2008[a]

((PDA$ or handheld$ or "personal digital assistant" or "personal digital assistants") and (nurs$ and education$)).mp. [mp = title, subject heading word, abstract, instrumentation]

Ovid MEDLINE 1950 to Week 4 March 2008[b]

((PDA$ or handheld$ or "personal digital assistant" or "personal digital assistants") and (nurs$ and education$)).mp. [mp = title, original title, abstract, name of substance word, subject heading word]

[a] University of Arizona Health Sciences Library.
[b] Arizona State University Libraries.

of required software onto it. Unfortunately, in these situations, it is difficult to allot time for teaching students how to use the PDA and there is typically no institutional technology support for problems that occur with the software or the hardware.[28,29,49,50] Managing large classes of students is extremely challenging under these circumstances.

Introducing PDAs into a program in all courses simultaneously (undergraduate, graduate, or both) requires detailed planning, but solves more problems than it creates. Schools have been successful in supporting large-scale introduction of PDAs into the curriculum by applying for a grant, expanding information technology budgets, or seeking a gift from a private donor or foundation.[12,19,23,32,34,50,51] This practice allows programs to build technology infrastructure to support the use of PDAs and to allot time for a critical mass of faculty, preceptors, and other stakeholders to learn to use the devices and software, to prepare PDA-centric learning exercises, and to model using PDAs in teaching and practice.[9,18–22,26–31,34,49,50,52–59] It also minimizes confusion over which students and courses are using PDAs and precludes students from feeling left out of a new initiative. Although many schools purchase PDAs for faculty and students in their initial implementation, their experiences suggest that schools should not purchase PDAs for either faculty or students. The devices' relatively short life spans do not make them a good investment for schools.[9,28–32,34,60] PDAs are sufficiently commonplace that students are not surprised to be required to purchase a specific PDA and are eager to be taught how to use it in clinical practice.[7,9,20] Making PDAs a program requirement allows students to use scholarship monies to purchase the devices, provides motivation for integrating PDAs into classroom and clinical studies, ensures that students will have late-model PDAs, and facilitates the transition of PDAs into clinical practice after graduation.

Lessons Learned about Hardware Adoption

To obtain volume discounts and to decrease the need for technology support, one device should be required for all students. Adoption decisions should be based on operating system capability (eg, Palm, Windows Mobile 6, Apple, Linux, Android), congruence with other university technology systems, availability of institutional technology support for students, faculty, and preceptors, quality of screen technology, type of connection technology (eg, Wi-Fi, Bluetooth, cell phone), availability of relevant software, volume discounts, and availability of sufficient numbers of devices.[17,20,52,54,55,57,58,60,61] Some consideration should be given to the short life span of devices that have been in the marketplace for more than a year. A decision to require a smartphone carries with it a monthly subscription bill, which is unlikely to be covered by scholarships. Additionally, PDA use, especially Wi-Fi and cell-phone connectivity, may be restricted by technology policies at practice sites where students are precepted.[10,12]

Lessons Learned about Software Adoption

Companies dedicated to producing health care software (eg, Skyscape, Lexi-Comp, Pepid, Epocrates, Unbound Medicine) provide their software on various hardware platforms and operating systems, including Palm, Windows Mobile 6, Symbian, Blackberry, and Apple. Software selection thus depends primarily on the level of education, prelicensure or graduate program, and faculty preferences,[10,11,51,60] rather than hardware. Choosing software that provides a digital version of reference textbooks that are already in use in the program minimizes transition cost and effort. Students should not be required to purchase a reference in more than one format, however. For instance, if a drug guide is going to be used, the student should purchase it for use on the PDA, for the desktop, or in the text form, but not in two or three forms unless the company is offering a steep discount for multiformat purchases. Students should also not be required to purchase references that duplicate content. For example, e-book versions of preferred textbooks may overlap completely with a publisher's suite of integrated PDA software. The contents of publishers' suites of software should be scrutinized carefully.

Although book publishers may offer their reference texts in a digital e-book format that can be used on a PDA, students, faculty, and clinicians do not read a reference text from cover to cover, typically. What makes texts useful on the PDA is conversion to a searchable format that is linked to other references on the device. For example, a diagnostic text should be linked to a laboratory values guide and a drug guide. In this way users can quickly obtain comprehensive answers to clinical questions.[62] Publishers accomplish this integration by specialty programming; thus each publisher's suite of programs functions differently. Care should be taken to choose suites that meet program needs.

Another method of reducing transition costs and effort is to limit the number of software programs that students, faculty, and preceptors must buy initially.[12,25,32,38,43,49] Requiring five to seven programs facilitates learning what these programs contain and how to use them. The typical suite should include a drug reference, a drug interaction guide, a laboratory reference, a disease reference, a medical dictionary, and a medical calculation program. Additional course-specific software (eg, health assessment and procedures manuals) and population-specific software (eg, pediatric, adult) can be added incrementally as each course is taught in the curriculum. This method spreads the cost of software over several semesters and ensures that the latest edition is being used. The frequency with which software on the PDA is updated is one of the real benefits to purchasing reference material in this format. Faculty should review their software recommendations regularly as they would traditional textbooks.

BACK TO THE FUTURE

The problem with the historical cycle of PDA use (see **Fig. 1**) is that improvements in PDA technology aimed at the generic consumer's personal use, rather than at creative ways to accomplish critical tasks, will not be transformational for nursing education and practice. These improvements will not be timely, efficient, or effective means to accomplish an objective, because the objective was not part of the development process. **Fig. 2** illustrates a model for maximizing the impact of PDAs on technological innovation in nursing education and practice.

Faculty must serve as the conduit between software/hardware developers and users (A in **Fig. 2**). Faculty are in the best position to articulate the current, future, and far-future needs of nursing, because they routinely interact in the clinical environment with preceptors, nurses, patients, and students.[7,34] They can ensure that innovations in PDA technology not only support the needs of health care professionals, but create previously unrecognized needs as users envision new solutions to unaddressed or newly encountered problems.[39,63] Developers are willing partners in this process, because evolving needs create increased demand for their products. Educational use drives implementation in the clinical setting, as graduates enter practice with PDAs in hand (B in **Fig. 2**). Use in educational and clinical settings enriches personal use (B and C in **Fig. 2**) and ensures that users provide feedback to educators about evolving needs for integrated solutions to clinical practice problems (D in **Fig. 2**).

This model supports several levels of technology use. In the lowest level, faculty use the PDA to help students manage information sources, such as standard nursing

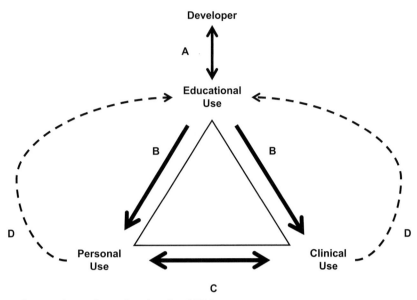

Fig. 2. Proposed transformational cycle of PDA use.

reference books, standardized practice guidelines, and medical calculation tools. Faculty and preceptors who go beyond this level use the PDA to encourage students to develop clinical logs and track patients, encounters, and procedures; consult laboratory, procedure, and pharmaceutical guides at the point of care; and pull information from evidence-based practice guidelines and reports of original research.[32,36,42,43,64–67] At the highest level, faculty use PDAs to nurture a habit of scientific and clinical inquiry by teaching students to pose questions and search for answers from e-reference books, PDA software that links reference materials to decision-making tools, and online databases of peer-reviewed journals.[7,25]

The primary barrier to implementation of the proposed model is the lack of a clearly articulated framework of technology innovation in nursing education. The typical implementation of technology in nursing education is a "back to the future" process. For example, when educators become aware that students are using PDAs for text messaging or podcasting, they try to make coursework more appealing by applying the technology. This process takes a traditional method of pedagogy and layers technology on top of it; for example, educators hold virtual office hours with students by way of e-mail, instant messaging, or Skype chats, or they begin podcasting or blogging supplemental material to push information to students. Although many of these efforts are enormously creative, they are inherently reactive and are often based on the assumption that knowledge is acquired formally and used statically. The technology may make the old way of doing business more appealing or more efficient, but it does not represent a novel way of teaching or using knowledge.

Using technology to transform education and practice requires more than layering technology onto instructional processes; it requires changing assumptions about knowledge acquisition and use.[39,63,68–70] For example, information retrieval should not be considered a static process. It is not enough for a student or clinician to download a pharmaceutical guide to the PDA and use it as a fact-checking device when prescribing. Innovative educators are attempting to transform the delivery of evidence-based health care with technologies that provide information at the point of decision; that is, they empower the clinician to pose a question, answer the question on the spot, and share the results with the patient. This method is based on the premise that answers to clinical questions exist in the "data cloud" and are readily accessible by students, faculty, and clinicians.[71]

In this framework, knowledge acquisition will be by means of data mining and knowledge use will take place in the moment in time when decisions need to be made. PDA technology will be a necessity to enable the clinician to be untethered. Educators will focus on stimulating systematic inquiry and critical thinking (ie, critical appraisal of the results of data mining). Selectivity, evaluation, and synthesis will be the hallmarks of information navigation and knowledge application.[69,70]

Today's undergraduates are natives of the digital world who exploit models of collaborative learning borrowed from online game play, simulated life, and social networks.[7,69,70] This concept is eloquently described by Andrea Saveri[68] "[They] practice cooperative and collective behaviors to augment their individual capabilities. What distinguishes them is their ability to use physical and digital spaces to activate their social networks and leverage the collective resource base to solve complex problems or catalyze collective action." Rather than going back to the future, educators will capitalize on the strengths of student networks and shape students' use of them to harness distributed intelligence in educational and clinical settings.[69,70] This use of distributed intelligence in collaborative communities will infuse goal-oriented innovation into nursing practice. Faculty, preceptors, and students will use existing technology to inspire ideas for better goal-oriented technology—technology that supports real-time evidence based practice.

REFERENCES

1. Wiggins RH III. Personal digital assistants. J Digit Imaging 2004;17(1):5–17.
2. Tooey MJ, Mayo A. Handheld technologies in a clinical setting: state of the technology and resources. AACN Clin Issues 2003;14(3):342–9.
3. Englebardt SP, Nelson R. Health care informatics. St. Louis (MO): Mosby; 2002.
4. Fishman SM. Palmtop computers on the medical wards. JAMA 1992;267(1):169.
5. Labkoff SE, Shah S, Bormel J, et al. The constellation project: experience and evaluation of personal digital assistants in the clinical environment. Proc Annu Symp Comput Appl Med Care 1995;19:678–82.
6. Lehman K. Clinical nursing instructors' use of handheld computers for student recordkeeping and evaluation. J Nurs Educ 2003;42(1):41–2.
7. Stroud SD, Erkel EA, Smith CA. The use of personal digital assistants by nurse practitioner students and faculty. J Am Acad Nurse Pract 2005;17(2):67–75.
8. Peterson M. The personal digital assistant and its future in nursing. Kans Nurse 2003;78(9):1–3.
9. Scollin P, Callahan J, Mehta A, et al. The PDA as a reference tool: libraries' role in enhancing nursing education. Comput Inform Nurs 2006;24(4):208–13.
10. Rosenthal K. Get "smart" with a PDA. Nurs Manage 2004;35(Suppl 5):17–8.
11. Rosenthal K. "Touch" vs. "tech": valuing nursing-specific PDA software. Nurs Manage 2003;34(7):58–60.
12. White A, Allen P, Goodwin L, et al. Infusing PDA technology into nursing education. Nurse Educ 2005;30(4):150–4.
13. Lewis JA, Sommers CO. Personal data assistants: using new technology to enhance nursing practice. American Journal of Maternal/Child Nursing 2003; 28(2):66–71.

14. Stern EA. Don't go to work without your backup brain! Comput Inform Nurs 2007; 25(5):258–63.
15. Kneebone R, Nestel D, Ratnasothy J, et al. The use of handheld computers in scenario-based procedural assessments. Med Teach 2003;25(6):632–42.
16. Bosma L, Balen RM, Davidson E, et al. Point of care use of a personal digital assistant for patient consultation management: experience of an intravenous resource nurse team in a major Canadian teaching hospital. Comput Inform Nurs 2003;21(4):179–85.
17. Shneyder Y. Personal digital assistants (PDA) for the nurse practitioner. J Pediatr Health Care 2002;16(6):317–20.
18. Giammattei FP. Implementing a total joint registry using personal digital assistants. A proof of concept. Orthop Nurs 2003;22(4):284–8.
19. Rust JE, Tafflinger T. Quality in your hands: using PDA technology for data collection. Clin Nurse Spec 2004;18(4):175–7.
20. Huffstutler S, Wyatt TH, Wright CP. The use of handheld technology in nursing education. Nurse Educ 2002;27(6):271–5.
21. Krauskopf PB, Wyatt TH. Even techno-phobic NPs can use PDAs. Nurse Pract 2006;31(7):48–52.
22. Krauskopf PB, Wyatt TH. Point counter-point: should NP students be encouraged to use PDAs during clinical learning experiences? Journal for Nurse Practitioners 2006;2(10):680–1.
23. Smith CM, Pattillo RE. PDAs in the nursing curriculum: providing data for internal funding. Nurse Educ 2006;31(3):101–2.
24. Fisher KL, Koren A. Palm perspectives: the use of personal digital assistants in nursing clinical education. A qualitative study. Online Journal of Nursing Informatics 2007;11(2) [online].
25. Pattillo RE, Brewer M, Smith CM. Tracking clinical use of personal digital assistant reference resources. Nurse Educ 2007;32(1):39–42.
26. Koeniger-Donohue R. Handheld computers in nursing education: a PDA pilot project. J Nurs Educ 2008;47(2):74–7.
27. Martin RR. Making a case for personal digital assistant (PDA) use in baccalaureate nursing education. Online Journal of Nursing Informatics 2007;11(2) [online].
28. Glasgow ME, Cornelius FH. Benefits and costs of integrating technology into undergraduate nursing programs. Nurs Leadersh Forum 2005;9(4):175–9.
29. Dreher HM, Cornelius F, Draper J, et al. The fusion of gerontology and technology in nursing education: history and demonstration of the gerontological informatics reasoning project–GRIP. Stud Health Technol Inform 2006;122:486–9.
30. Cornelius F, Donnelly GF. Point of care technology to enhance student learning and patient outcomes: Drexel University's PDA initiative. Deans Notes 2006; 27(3):1–2.
31. Cornelius F, Gordon MG. Introducing and using handheld technology in nursing education. Annual Review of Nursing Education 2006;4:179–92.
32. Altmann TK, Brady D. PDAs bring information competence to the point-of-care. Int J Nurs Educ Scholarsh 2005;2(1):1–14.
33. Honeybourne C, Sutton S, Ward L. Knowledge in the palm of your hands: PDAs in the clinical setting. Health Info Libr J 2006;23(1):51–9.
34. Scollin P, HealeyWalsh J, Kafel K, et al. Evaluating students' attitudes to using PDAs in nursing clinicals at two schools. Comput Inform Nurs 2007;25(4):228–35.
35. Greenfield S. Medication error reduction and the use of PDA technology. J Nurs Educ 2007;46(3):127–31.

36. Trangenstein P, Weiner E, Gordon J, et al. Data mining results from an electronic clinical log for nurse practitioner students. Medinfo 2007;12(Pt 2):1387–91.
37. Currie LM, Desjardins KS, Stone PW, et al. Near-miss and hazard reporting: promoting mindfulness in patient safety education. Medinfo 2007;12(Pt 1):285–90.
38. Carlton KH, Dillard N, Campbell BR, et al. Personal digital assistants for classroom and clinical use. Comput Inform Nurs 2007;25(5):253–8.
39. Momtahan KL, Burns CM, Sherrard H, et al. Using personal digital assistants and patient care algorithms to improve access to cardiac care best practices. Medinfo 2007;12(Pt 1):117–21.
40. Lee T, Lin K, Lin J. Development and testing of an evaluation scale of personal digital assistants. Comput Inform Nurs 2007;25(3):171–9.
41. Lee NJ, Bakken S. Preliminary analysis for the development of a PDA-based decision support system for the screening and management of obesity. Stud Health Technol Inform 2006;122:129–33.
42. Bakken S, Jenkins M, Choi J, et al. Usefulness of a personal digital assistant-based advanced practice nursing student clinical log: faculty stakeholder exemplars. Stud Health Technol Inform 2006;122:698–702.
43. Garrett BM, Jackson C. A mobile clinical e-portfolio for nursing and medical students, using wireless personal digital assistants (PDAs). Nurse Educ Today 2006; 26(8):647–54.
44. Farrell M. Nursing and midwifery education using mobile technologies. Aust Nurs J 2006;14(1):25.
45. Farrell MJ, Rose L. Use of mobile handheld computers in clinical nursing education. J Nurs Educ 2008;47(1):13–9.
46. John R, Buschman P, Chaszar M, et al. Development and evaluation of a PDA-based decision support system for pediatric depression screening. Medinfo 2007;12(Pt 2):1382–6.
47. Kerkenbush NL, Lasome CE. The emerging role of electronic diaries in the management of diabetes mellitus. AACN Clin Issues 2003;14(3):371–8.
48. Kho A, Henderson LE, Dressler DD, et al. Use of handheld computers in medical education. A systematic review. J Gen Intern Med 2006;21(5):531–7.
49. Colevins H, Bond D, Clark K. Nurse refresher students get a hand from handhelds. Computer in Libraries 2006;26(4):6–8, 46–8.
50. Tilghman J, Raley D, Conway JJ. Family nurse practitioner students' utilization of personal digital assistants (PDAs): implications for practice. ABNF J 2006;17(3): 115–7.
51. Blair R. Take-along tech and the training of specialty nurses. Health Manag Technol 2006;27(3):44, 46–7.
52. Miller J, Shaw-Kokot JR, Arnold MS, et al. A study of personal digital assistants to enhance undergraduate clinical nursing education. J Nurs Educ 2005;44(1): 19–26.
53. Nacey G. The human touch. Health Manag Technol 2007;(7):39–40.
54. Ndiwane A. Teaching with the Nightingale tracker technology in community-based nursing education: a pilot study. J Nurs Educ 2005;44(1):40–2.
55. Newman K, Howse E. The impact of a PDA-assisted documentation tutorial on student nurses' attitudes. Comput Inform Nurs 2007;25(2):76–83.
56. Berglund M, Nilsson C, Revay P, et al. Nurses' and nurse students' demands of functions and usability in a PDA. Int J Med Inf 2007;76(7):530–7.
57. Scordo KA, Yeager S, Young L. Use of personal digital assistants with acute care nurse practitioner students. AACN Clin Issues 2003;14(3):350–62.

58. Sloan HL, Delahoussaye CP. Clinical application of the Omaha system with the Nightingale tracker: a community health nursing student home visit program. Nurse Educ 2003;28(1):15–7.
59. Utterback K, Waldo BH. Matching point-of-care devices to clinicians for positive outcomes. Home Healthc Nurse 2005;23(7):452–61.
60. Hunt EC. The value of a PDA to a nurse. Tar Heel Nurse 2002;64(3):18–9.
61. Bower NS. Put technology at your fingertips with a PDA. Nurse Pract 2004;29(2): 45–6.
62. McCord G, Smucker WD, Selius BA, et al. Answering questions at the point of care: do residents practice EBM or manage information sources? Acad Med 2007;82:298–303.
63. Momtahan K, Burns C. Applications of ecological interface design in supporting the nursing process. J Healthc Inf Manag 2004;18(4):74–82.
64. Grady M, Yates VM. Portable media players in the skills laboratory. Nurs Educ Perspect 2007;28(2):62–3.
65. Smith-Stoner M. 10 uses for personal digital assistants in home care. Home Healthc Nurse 2003;21(12):797–800.
66. Maag M. Podcasting and MP3 players: emerging education technologies. Comput Inform Nurs 2006;24(1):9–13.
67. Stoten S. Using podcasts for nursing education. J Contin Educ Nurs 2007;38(2): 56–7.
68. Saveri A. The Cybernomadic framework. SR-843. Menlo Park (CA): Institute for the Future; 2004.
69. Brown JS, Adler RP. Minds of fire: open education, the long tail, and learning 2.0. Educause Review 2008;43(1):17–32.
70. Brown JS. New learning environments for the 21st century: exploring the edge. Change 2006;38(5):18–24.
71. Hargraves O. The data cloud. Language Lounge. Available at: http://www.visualthesaurus.com/cm/ll/1331/. Accessed March 1, 2008.

The Use of Simulation Technology in the Education of Nursing Students

Maria Overstreet, PhD(c), RN, CCNS

KEYWORDS

- Simulation • High-fidelity • Nursing • Education • Scenario
- Critical thinking

Nursing education historically has used an education model that includes the use of reading and lecture for knowledge gain, the laboratory setting for hand-eye coordination or psychomotor skill development, and the clinical setting with live patients for the practice of combining knowledge, psychomotor skill, and decision making at the bedside. An apprenticeship model for health care education remained intact until the late 1960s when an alternative for medical anesthesia residents came to life. With the advent of "Sim One," a computer-controlled mannequin created by Abrahamson and Denson,[1,2] anesthesia residents soon began to practice the skill of intubation on the mannequin. This practice was the beginning of advanced skill teaching with the use of a responsive mannequin with the intent to increase the proficiency and accuracy of student performance. Since then, simulation use in health care education has grown. Simulation is not a new teaching tool; nurse educators have used role play and static mannequins to simulate patient situations for decades. What is new is advanced computer technology allowing simulation to be even more lifelike. Simulation as defined for this article includes exercises for the learner that represent lifelike situations in a health care setting including a computer driven mannequin patient that is responsive to a learner's intervention. The purpose of this article is to provide historical and foundational knowledge about simulation, educational theory, current research efforts in the use of simulation in health care, and application of nursing clinical simulation guided by theory and research.

SIMULATION IN THE PRESENT

Simulation computer technology has evolved from an entire room of computers managed by multiple highly trained personnel to a more economical and user-friendly

Vanderbilt School of Nursing, 303 Godchaux Hall, 461 21st Avenue South, Nashville, TN 37240, USA
E-mail address: maria.overstreet@vanderbilt.edu

Nurs Clin N Am 43 (2008) 593–603
doi:10.1016/j.cnur.2008.06.009
0029-6465/08/$ – see front matter
nursing.theclinics.com

personal computer. With this evolution of the hardware and software required for simulation, educators began to envision how to use this tool to assist the learner, thus producing simulation exercises. Simulation spread quickly in the medical community and within the past 10 years nurse educators and nurse researchers have become increasingly intrigued. Is this new technology here to stay? This question remains unanswered; however, researchers have begun to explore the use of simulation and how simulation can best be used as a teaching tool in health care education. See **Table 1** for a summary of simulation research that includes sentinel articles. After careful review of nursing, medicine, and education literature on simulation, there are more than 2000 articles, which include commentaries to true experimental studies and which range from evaluation of individual performance to team performance and evaluation of the acquisition of skills, such as knowledge, psychomotor, self confidence, self efficacy, and communication. More recent studies have been designed to investigate the critical thinking and decision-making aspects simulation may offer, such as how students may use simulation to learn to prioritize care and make decisions at the point of care. Various contexts also are being created in simulation to assist students in preparing for future decision-making roles related to terrorism, such as exercises in mass casualty or exposure to toxic agents as a health care provider.[17,18] Simulation exercises such as these can theoretically assist the learner to be in an unfamiliar place and encounter the knowledge component, the psychomotor skills, and the decision-making capabilities of caring for the patient, family, or community.

Simulation exercises also can recreate the emotional environment for the learner,[19] a skill a learner may seldom have the opportunity to practice. These exercises can provide the learner a safe place to practice his or her reaction to a particular emotionally charged experience. Besides experiencing the knowledge component, the psychomotor skill development, and the critical thinking aspects to simulation the learner also may experience the emotional, spiritual, and ethical components of providing care to patients and families, ideas studied in the context of nursing simulation.[20] Learners may engage in a simulation exercise that offers the specific objective of learning how to work with the feelings of patients, family members, peers, and themselves when a patient dies. Experiencing an emotional component while learning can help to store new information for recall later.[19,21] Place yourself in the shoes of a nursing student who has never witnessed a patient dying, or has never experienced working with a patient suffering the merciless pain of pancreatic cancer or the patient who lost her baby at birth. These situations are life's dilemmas, an emotionally charged environment where nurses work day after day. Simulation exercises offer learners the opportunity to experience the atmosphere, the setting, the feelings, the emotion, the smells, and most importantly, their own reactions to health care dilemmas patients and families encounter. The simulated environment allows learners to begin to formulate how they will respond. The learner then has the opportunity to practice his or her words, actions, and reactions in a repetitive fashion if so desired.

Recent growth in the area of simulations for nursing education has resulted in a new organization called the International Nursing Association for Clinical Simulation and Learning (www.inacsl.org). Besides sponsoring an annual conference, the group also hosts a listserv for e-mail and an online journal.

EDUCATIONAL THEORY

Nursing education is rooted in experiential learning theory, a hands-on approach to education. Dewey's theory of experiential learning[21] posits that when a learner becomes engaged in the doing or the performance, learning may occur. Apprenticeships are an example of an early form of experiential learning in which the learner observes and performs the actual work under the guidance of a master teacher. It is through these guided hands-on experiences that the memory of events, actions, and even words are formed that the learner stores and can return to or draw from in future situations.

Simulation exercises are hands-on experiential learning. The learner has the opportunity to observe, to do, to practice, and to experience. Simulation is thus rooted in Dewey's theory of experiential learning. In an attempt to explain experiential learning Dewey offers the example of a young child learning about fire and the consequences of getting too close to the fire. The child may have no experience to reflect on that offers the awareness of consequences to touching the fire.[21] The child may thus learn by experience that standing too close to the fire hurts or burns. Awareness of consequences from previous experiences is a part of experiential learning. For example, if a student nurse has no experience in working with intensive care patients receiving mechanical ventilation, there is no memory of consequences from which to draw. An experienced nurse may automatically know how to work with a certain patient situation because either they experienced it before or can interpret another experience and relate it to a similar principle. The novice nursing student has no experience to reference. Simulation can create the opportunity for the student nurse to gain these experiences to be called on in future practice.

In addition to Dewey's theory of experiential learning, Kolb[22] describes a learning cycle that he believes helps to visualize how an adult learner processes experiential learning. Kolb posits that the learner enters the cycle at a point that is most comfortable to his or her learning style: concrete or abstract. The next dichotomy is the use of reflection versus experimentation, both of which are continuations of experiential learning. The nursing clinical simulation described through Kolb's cycle of learning (**Fig. 1**) was designed to bring Kolb's cycle of learning to a more concrete or testable level with nursing clinical simulation. The learner may have completed the hands-on portion of the simulation without much learning; however, during the debriefing the learner may discover a concept never considered before and begin formulating how to test this new concept. A repeat simulation might be the most appropriate next step for the learner, which would be consistent with experiential learning theory; however, the practical answer for today's nurse educator may be for the learner to use a different form of experiential learning, simulated computer gaming, which one can do alone for reinforcement or practice of skills or decision making.

So, how does a learner take the experience of learning and make sense of it or apply the same principles to another situation? Schön's theory of reflective practice[23] offers the educator a base on which to assist learners in making sense of their experiences. Schön posits that to gain purpose in our actions we must be able to perform self-reflection. Typically, following a simulation exercise, the educator facilitates a debriefing experience for the learners. The purpose of the debriefing is to assist the learners to make sense of their experience, to reflect on their actions, and to gain insight to their emotions. Reflection in action (during the simulation exercise) and reflection on action (following the simulation exercise), as described by Schön, allows learners to become more aware of their responses.[23] Building more self-reflective capabilities allows students to become more aware of their actions and reactions and able to identify when they need to change a behavior, attitude, or other skill set. The debriefing time also allows learners a time to vocalize their feelings and emotions about a specific act, thus placing more emphasis on the learner's ability to create or recreate a memory store or solidify the experience.[19,21]

Table 1
Simulation research results

Author	Area of Concentration	Results
Waldner[3]	Theory to experience for nursing students	Describe through Benner's and Kolb's theories the use of simulation to support nursing student transition; theory to practice.
Wellard[4]	Explored current use of clinical laboratory practices in Australia	Wondered why education in laboratory taught certain topics. Discovered laboratory learning was based on tradition, not best practices.
Lasater[5]	Qualitative study of nursing students' development of clinical judgment	Used focus groups to study the development of clinical judgment. Simulation forced learning to anticipate what might happen. Heightened awareness in clinical setting. Debriefing improved reflection.
Radhakrishnan[6]	Pilot study: measure clinical practice parameters with HPS	Attempt to evaluate effects of simulation practice on the clinical performance of 12 BSN students. Five areas identified by faculty, one sensitive to simulation: safety.
Scherer[7]	Nurse practitioner student knowledge and confidence	Pilot study: 23 subjects, randomly assigned, pre- and posttest knowledge and confidence. No difference in knowledge tests scores. Control group scored significantly higher posttest confidence ($P = .040$).
Bradley[8]	History of simulation in medical education	Discussion of theory and research and future directions of simulation and factors driving the use of simulation in health care.
Rudolph[9]	Debriefing and judgment	Share approach to debriefing emphasizing good judgment.
Ziv[10]	Cultural change in medical education	Presents "error-driven" educational approach in simulation-based medical education; highlights lessons learned.
Klein[11]	Use simulation as primary means of evaluating learning	Used COPA model to redesign curriculum and used simulation to evaluate nursing student learning.
McCausland[12]	Provides guide to others ready to embark on simulation	Provides important lessons learned through experience with simulation and guides to those beginning a simulation program.
Howard[13]	Sleep deprivation effects on psychomotor and clinical performance	Used simulation to study rested versus sleep-deprived anesthesiologists. Psychomotor performance and mood were impaired.

(*continued on next page*)

Author	Area of Concentration	Results
Table 1 *(continued)*		
Gaba[14]	Compare and contrast two examples of how to evaluate impact of a new approach to teaching.	For a skill-specific task, use a checklist and view the videotape. If evaluating the value of the intervention must include multiple factors, not easily identifiable: financial, target, population, and goal.
Seymour[15]	Does the training of skills from virtual reality simulation transfer to operating room performance	Scored eight predefined errors for each procedure.Interrater reliability >0.080; 16 residents randomly assigned. Virtual reality simulation significantly improved residents' performance of laparoscopic cholecystectomy.
Bell[16]	Effect of simulation on anxiety	Pretest/posttest experimental design looked at anxiety of nursing student learning new psychomotor skill. (Not high-fidelity simulation but used same educational principles). Anxiety decreased when performing skill for first time with simulation versus real patient. Two groups did not differ in performance.

Simulation provides the medium in which to practice and reflect. The technology allows for the realism of the context of the situation with the added response from the patient and consequence of performed actions. Regardless of the sophistication of the technology it is still a tool. The debriefing allows a time for the educator to facilitate the learner's reflection on the experience and to make sense of the learning. The educator remains the most vital role in the dynamics of the experience for the learner.

The workload for creating, implementing, and redesigning simulations can be great. Continued research effort is needed in this particular sense of nursing clinical simulations to make sure this is an efficient and worthwhile use of faculty and student time.

APPLICATION OF NURSING CLINICAL SIMULATION GUIDED BY THEORY AND RESEARCH

The following is an example of my experience using educational theorists, Dewey, Kolb, and Schön, to guide the experience of simulation and using research to support concepts of nursing medication administration. The creation of this simulation is delineated in the following four phases:

Concepts: How I began
Theory: To guide my educational practice
Nuts and bolts: Putting it together
Debriefing: Trying out a new rhythm

Phase 1. Concepts: How I Began

Following careful review of the literature on nursing medication errors and discussion with Barbara Olson, RNC, BSN, MS, Safe Medication Management Fellow with the Institute for Safe Medication Practices (ISMP), I decided on the following concepts to provide in a simulation experience for nursing students: preparation and administration of

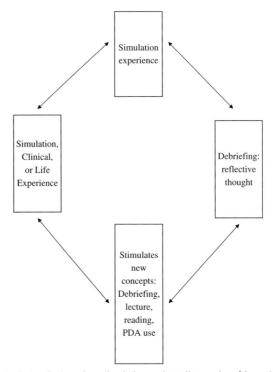

Fig. 1. Nursing clinical simulation described through Kolb's cycle of learning.

insulin and discovery of embedded system error. After much thought about these two related concepts, which are inherent in the work life of nurses, I knew if I could create a simulation challenging enough but not overwhelming, the nursing student might have the opportunity to experience discovering a system error or performing an actual error in a protected learning environment safe from patient harm. At this point, I asked myself if it was best for the student to perform an error and learn how it can happen or if it was better for the student to learn how system errors could lead to potential error at the patient's bedside. Again, after much debate and conversation with ISMP fellow Olson, I decided either experience would be a grand learning opportunity for any student. The concepts of medication error and system error were merged and the experiential learning format was chosen for a more hands-on, active learning process.

Phase 2. Theory: to Guide My Educational Practice

Why choose experiential learning? I have seen firsthand how nursing students respond to lecture, practice in the skills laboratory, and clinical experience with live patients. Now I also sport a few years of experience with nursing clinical simulations. What a grand opportunity I have to watch learning as it occurs. In lecture, there is not much time for discussion of issues, to bat back and forth ideas and alternatives. The learner is in a passive mode, attempting to accept this information and remember every word. My stance does not mean that lecture is worthless. I greatly believe one-way lecture has its place in health care education. There is a tremendous amount of facts nursing students have to know and memorize. Lecture and independent reading are acceptable educational methods of this type of knowledge dissemination. What

I wanted the student to learn, however, was more in the line of the type of learning that occurs in clinical or experiential learning. In the clinical experience, a major focus is on patient safety. The instructor and the bedside nurse consciously create a large safety net for the patient. The student must check and verify medications with either the instructor or the bedside nurse, which protects patient and student from error. In nursing clinical simulation, situations can be created to offer the student the experience of error. There is controversy as to whether simulation should be used as a platform for error discovery. Some argue that only best practices should be embedded to serve as positive role models for students. I believe, however, that the student deserves the opportunity to experience an error in a safe environment at least once for several reasons: to know what it feels like to have been at the delivery end of error, to discover how systems can fail, and to view the error from the patient's viewpoint. You will have to decide how to handle this situation in your simulations.

Phase 3. Nuts and Bolts: Putting it Together

After deciding on concepts and methods, I then began to hammer out the objectives for the learner during the experience. The realism of this scenario was a must. The learner must believe the patient is there and requiring his or her insulin medication. Support for all patient parameters, care required, and medications to deliver or not deliver stemmed from my nursing experience coupled with best practice guidelines. Do your research. Ask for involvement in this part of the development process by lecturers of the content or clinical instructors. Develop all your sources of information systematically and make notes. When you begin to implement the simulation and discover questions about content, you can find your sources quickly and remedy any out-of-date information or new evidence in the field. Also, if this turns out to be a simulation you want to continue to use, you will be able to adapt it quickly to new advances in the field if you keep a good tracking system of your notes.

An important aspect of simulation development is to pilot test the simulation with volunteer faculty and students. You may find you need to adjust some of the verbal content of the patient depending on the paths some faculty and students take. Have more than enough verbal recordings for as many imaginable routes as the simulation may take, unless of course you decide to provide the vocals yourself, on-the-fly or during the simulation exercise.

Next, if you are not currently in practice, I suggest a field trip. Go to the units where the students practice. Talk with the nurses on the patient care units and discuss your ideas of how medication errors happen in the simulation you have created. Make sure these are some of the errors the nurses have seen or heard of occurring today. Remember, equipment is expensive and realism is a must. You must sometimes make your choices within budgetary constraints while at the same time trying to achieve realistic effects. There are websites of organizations in nursing simulation where you can learn about how to create certain bodily fluids. You also can learn other tricks of the trade in simulation. You may want your students to sign a confidentiality agreement before the simulation. I decided to have the students sign this agreement. Basically, the students and I agree:

Simulation is a learning situation and learning is the primary objective.
What happens in simulation stays in simulation (this pertains to the keys of the simulation and to student behaviors).
Students know it is simulation and I know it is simulation and we will all treat it as real as possible.
Mistakes can be made in simulation and no patient is harmed.

Phase 4. Debriefing: Trying out a New Rhythm

Debriefing has been called the "heart and soul"[24] of simulation, the "crucial"[25] point of learning. Debriefing has many types of connotations that require faculty to select a type appropriate for their simulation session. The term itself is misunderstood and misrepresented in the literature, however. Debriefing comes from the military with the first known debriefing to occur as a result of Brigadier General Marshall, an army historian, trying to learn as much as he could about the combat situation.[26] Marshall would have groups of soldiers get together and discuss the events of the battlefield in as much detail as they could remember. Marshall noted an unexpected event at the end of the discussion: the soldiers seemed to feel better, which he called "spiritual purging."[27]

Another type of debriefing comes more from the psychology literature and is referred to as critical incident stress debriefing (CISD). This system of debriefing was created by Mitchell[28] as a brief form of counseling following a traumatic event. Today, CISD continues in use especially with health care responders to traumatic events.

There is scant literature concerning the debriefing phase of simulation. Opinion articles are abundant that refer to the debriefing phase as a pivotal point in the learning from simulation exercises. The attention paid to the process is brief, however. Gaba and colleagues[25] describe the goals for the learner during their debriefing process in an anesthesia simulation as threefold: explore alternatives, recognize principles that did and did not work, and link behaviors to the real world.

In a seminal study about the value of debriefing, Savoldelli and colleagues[29] used a control group who received no debriefing to compare against two experimental groups receiving either a verbal or a verbal plus video debriefing. These researchers discovered what several have believed about debriefing but never verified: debriefing is important. Using debriefing following a simulation exercise also allows for other teachable moments to emerge. The point of which method to use may depend on what type of simulation the learner experienced. If the learner had an emotional experience, the facilitator may choose to use more of a CISD approach.

Rudolph and colleagues[9] describe their form of reflective practice in health care simulation debriefing. They discuss debriefing with good judgment, a technique that includes the facilitator's observations and experienced opinion delivered in a respective manner to assist the learner in discovering the frames or mental model that drove his or her action.[9] This practice is theory driven. This type of debriefing is reflective of Schön's theory of reflective practice in that the question arises as to what drove the actions, discovering the frames of the learner. These educators have used this technique in more than 2000 debriefings and state they often found their own self-reflection and behavior changes in the trainees was encouraged.

Before choosing how you will debrief, it would be helpful to read Rudolph and colleagues,[9] Gaba and colleagues,[25] and other educational articles on debriefing by Lederman,[30] Pearson and Smith,[31] and Schön.[23] The type of debriefing I chose was a mixture of Schön, Rudolph, and Pearson and Smith. I created specific learner objectives for the simulation; however, I was flexible. What emerged as most important to the learner during the debriefing also was included. The order in which the debriefing occurred was driven by the learner. If the learner was emotionally moved by the experience, the debriefing of the feelings took priority. By using a method of conversation to debrief, learned from Rudolph and colleagues,[9] I facilitated the debriefing sessions with minimal input from my verbal self. This technique takes time to learn; however, it can be powerful when mastered. The learner is facilitated without evening knowing learning is in process. Emotions are released, concepts are discussed, critiques are given, and frames are discovered.

I learned as much as my students by participating in the simulation and debriefing process. As the simulation progressed, I learned how to gently tweak the realism as offered by participants. With each debriefing, there were similarities and differences. I discovered concepts to report back to lecturers and clinical instructors that most students did not understand, not for failure of their listening or failure of the lecturer of covering the material, but for failure of identifying better, more optimal ways for students to learn.

SIMULATION IN THE FUTURE

Best educational practices in the use of simulations are just now beginning to be shared. Are we using simulation with best educational practices in place? Are the simulation facilitators practicing the debriefing with good judgment?[9] These questions remain unanswered. Can educators determine the ethical practice of students by way of simulation exercises? Can educators assist students to encounter ethical situations in health care before working with patients? Will simulated learning carry over or transfer to clinical practice?

Longitudinal studies are needed to look at the practice of new graduates who have been educated with and without simulation embedded in the curriculum. A major focus area for nurse educators to consider in the use of simulation is the culture of safety for the patient and the nursing student. There are no studies that demonstrate if nursing simulation practice transfers to nursing clinical practice. Nurse researchers are in the early stages of the development of the body of knowledge needed to advance the science. We must be rigorous in our development of sound research in an attempt to validate a new teaching tool and best educational practices.

SUMMARY

The high fidelity equipment used in health care simulations can be exciting for the learner and the instructor. As nurse educators and nurse scientists, we must realize the multiple confounding variables that exist in simulation and be diligent in interpreting data from such studies. The next steps in nursing clinical simulation research are extremely important ones in developing the science further. Nursing clinical simulation debriefing is at a beginning point of research. Nursing must look to other disciplines using simulation and debriefing, review their uses, theories, evaluations, and student responses, and look toward outcomes, such as improved end-user data, that with nursing might include safer patient care through becoming a more deliberate, reflecting practitioner.

ACKNOWLEDGMENT

The author acknowledges the support and insight of Elizabeth E. Weiner, PhD, RN, BC, FAAN, Senior Associate Dean for Informatics at Vanderbilt University School of Nursing and Marian Roman, PhD, APRN, BC, Assistant Professor of Nursing, The University of Tennessee.

REFERENCES

1. Sinz E. Anesthesiology national CME program and ASA activities in simulation [Electronic version]. Anesthesiol Clin 2007;25:209–23.
2. Cooper J, Taqueti V. A brief history of the development of mannequin simulators for clinical education and training [Electronic version]. Qual Saf Health Care 2004; 13:11–8.

3. Waldner M, Olson J. Taking the patient to the classroom: applying theoretical frameworks to simulation in nursing education [Electronic version]. Int J Nurs Educ Scholarsh 2007;4(1):1–14.

4. Wellard S, Woolf R, Gleeson L. Exploring the use of clinical laboratories in undergraduate nursing programs in regional Australia. Int J Nurs Educ Scholarsh 2007; 4(1):1–11.

5. Lasater K. High-fidelity simulation and the development of clinical judgment: students' experiences [Electronic version]. J Nurs Educ 2007;46(6):269–76.

6. Radhakrishnan K, Roche J, Cunningham H. Measuring clinical practice parameters with human patient simulation: a pilot study [Electronic version]. Int J Nurs Educ Scholarsh 2007;4:Article 8.

7. Scherer Y, Bruce S, Runkawatt V. A comparison of clinical simulation and case study presentation on nurse practitioner students' knowledge and confidence in managing a cardiac event [Electronic version]. Int J Nurs Educ Scholarsh 2007;4(1):1–14.

8. Bradley P. The history of simulation in medical education and possible future directions [Electronic version]. Med Educ 2006;40:254–62.

9. Rudolph J, Simon R, Dufresne, et al. There's no such thing as "nonjudgmental" debriefing: a theory and method of debriefing with good judgment. Simulation in Healthcare 2006;1(1):49–55.

10. Ziv A, Erez D, Munz Y, et al. The Israel center for medical simulation: a paradigm for cultural change in medical education [Electronic version]. Acad Med 2006; 81(12):1091–7.

11. Klein C. Linking competency-based assessment to successful clinical practice [Electronic version]. J Nurs Educ 2006;45(9):379–83.

12. McCausland L, Curran C, Cataldi P. Use of a human simulator for undergraduate nurse education [Electronic version]. Int J Nurs Educ Scholarsh 2004;1(1):1–17.

13. Howard S, Gaba D, Smith B, et al. Simulation study of rested versus sleep-deprived anesthesiologists. [Electronic version]. Anesthesiology 2003;98:1345–55.

14. Gaba D. Two examples of how to evaluate the impact of new approaches to teaching [Electronic version]. Anesthesiology 2002;96(1):1–3.

15. Seymour N, Gallagher A, Roman S, et al. Virtual reality training improves operating room performance [Electronic version]. Ann Surg 2002;236(4):458–64.

16. Bell M. 1986. Learning a complex nursing skill: student anxiety and the effect of simulated skill evaluation. The University of Texas at Austin, Dissertation. Accession No: AAG8618419.

17. Doran A, Mulhall M. Bioterrorism in the simulation laboratory: preparing students for the unexpected [Electronic version]. J Nurs Educ 2007;46(6):292.

18. Scott J, Miller G, Issenberg B, et al. Skill improvement during emergency response to terrorism training [Electronic version]. Prehosp Emerg Care 2006; 10:507–14.

19. Lammers R. Simulation: the new teaching tool [Electronic version]. Ann Emerg Med 2007;49(4):505–7.

20. Spunt D, Foster D, Adams K. Mock code: a clinical simulation module [Electronic version]. Nurs Educ 2004;29(5):192–4.

21. Dewey J. Experience and education. New York: Macmillian; 1938.

22. Kolb D. Experiential learning: experience as the source of learning and development. New Jersey (NJ): Prentice Hall; 1984.

23. Schön D. Educating the reflective practitioner. San Francisco (CA): Jossey-Bass; 1987.

24. Rall M, Manser T, Howard S. Key elements of debriefing for simulator training [Electronic version]. Eur J Anaesthesiol 2000;17(8):516–7.
25. Gaba D, Howard S, Fish K, et al. Simulation-based training in anesthesia crisis resource management (ACRM): a decade of experience [Electronic version]. Simul Gaming 2001;32(2):175–93.
26. Fillion J, Clements P, Averill J, et al. Talking as a primary method of peer defusing for military personnel exposed to combat trauma [Electronic version]. J Psychosoc Nurs Ment Health Serv 2002;40(8):40–9.
27. MacDonald C. Evaluation of stress debriefing interventions with military populations [Electronic version]. Mil Med 2003;168(12):961–8.
28. Mitchell J. When disaster strikes…the critical incident stress debriefing process [Electronic version]. Journal of Emergency Medical Services 1983;8(1):36–9.
29. Savoldelli G, Nalk V, Park J, et al. Value of debriefing during simulated crisis management: oral versus video-assisted oral feedback [Electronic version]. Anesthesiology 2006;105(2):279–85.
30. Lederman L. Debriefing: a critical reexamination of the postexperience analytic process with implications for its effective use [Electronic version]. Simul Games 1984;15(4):415–31.
31. Pearson M, Smith D. Debriefing in experience-based learning. Simulation/games for Learning 1986;16(4):155–72.

Developing the Online Survey

Jeffry S. Gordon, PhD*, Ryan McNew, AAS, CNE

KEYWORDS

- Email data collection • Web-based survey
- Personal digital assistant

The growing popularity of the Internet beginning in the mid-1990s has made it much easier for survey makers to administer their data collection tools to a much greater audience. Until that time, surveys were administered face to face, by telephone, through "snail" mail, or at response centers.[1] All of these methods were expensive (staffing, postage, printing, and envelope stuffing) and inconvenient.[2] With the invention of the Internet and its attending software tools, survey deployment suddenly became much cheaper and efficient.[3]

This article discusses various approaches to using the Internet for survey style data collection and the pro's and con's of each approach and outlines several issues one must consider when creating online survey instruments. For the purposes of this article, a "survey" is defined as any online tool that collects data. From the computer's perspective, any software that implements a form object such as a text entry box, radio button, dropdown choices, checkboxes, or graphics hotspots to collect data is a survey. By this definition, an electronic medical record system is a survey. E-commerce applications are surveys. In fact, any application that asks for any information to be put into an electronic document is, from the computer's perspective, a survey.

The authors assume that the reader already understands the basic tenets of proper survey design. All of the correct practices in question development and organization also apply to its online counterpart.[4] Although there are additional design considerations for a 17-in color monitor and a device capable of branching logic, the basic concepts in paper survey construction apply to online surveys as well.

There are three basic approaches to collecting data online. The first is through e-mail,[1] the second is through the Web,[1] and the third is through personal digital assistants (PDAs) or handheld devices.

E-MAIL DATA COLLECTION

Early in the 1990s, e-mail became a primary method of communication. With an e-mail distribution list, it was possible to send an e-mail to a list of potential responders and

School of Nursing, Vanderbilt University, 461 21st Avenue South, Nashville, TN 37240, USA
* Corresponding author.
E-mail address: jeff.s.gordon@vanderbilt.edu (J.S. Gordon).

Nurs Clin N Am 43 (2008) 605–619
doi:10.1016/j.cnur.2008.06.011
0029-6465/08/$ – see front matter © 2008 Elsevier Inc. All rights reserved.

attach a word-processed file containing a questionnaire. The respondent would detach the attachment from the e-mail, fill out the survey using whatever word processing tool they happened to have handy, save the file back, and send the attachment in a new e-mail back to the original sender. This technique is still in use today. Although it works well with a small intimate sample, the procedure is fraught with issues and problems.

On the positive side, the procedure is easy to implement. The primary technical skills of the sender include how to create the question file in Word or Acrobat, how to attach the file to an e-mail, and how to send the file through a distribution list such as Outlook or a list created in Listserv or MajorDomo. The responder has to know how to detach the attachment from the e-mail, fill out the form, save it, attach it to a responding e-mail, and send it back.

Although e-mail may be easy, it is not without serious issues and concerns. First, e-mail is not anonymous. When the person replies to the survey, their identity is known through their e-mail address.[5] Research indicates that some people respond differently if they know they are identifiable. Second, some e-mail servers block incoming e-mails with ".doc" as an extension on file attachments. In short, the e-mail gets treated by the e-mail server as spam and is either relegated to a spam folder or deleted outright.[5] To get around this problem, the survey creator can send the survey in an Adobe Acrobat PDF format, but this requires the sender to own and know how to use Adobe Acrobat Writer and for the respondent to have a PDF reader on their machine that is capable of reading the file. Furthermore, the end user will have to be able to write back into the file itself and send it back. Finally, there is the problem of transcribing the data from the Word or PDF form into a data device area such as an Access database application. Transcription not only is expensive but also allows for typographical errors to creep into the dataset.[6] Although sending surveys through e-mail is very doable for even the techno novice, it is not an acceptable approach for the reasons already outlined. Nevertheless, small informal surveys with respondents who do not care about lack of anonymity can use this approach. The e-mail approach can often be used to pilot test a survey to see if the survey is constructed correctly and is asking the right questions.

WEB-BASED SURVEYS

There are many benefits to creating a survey on a Web site. First, the response can be relatively anonymous. Although it is possible for the survey to grab the respondent's Internet protocol (IP) address, going any further to identify the person would require a court order; therefore, anonymity is fairly well preserved. Second, the data can be automatically stored inside a database for later data mining and analysis. Because the data go in "automatically," there is no chance of introducing typographical errors that occur during transcription. In addition, transcription costs are nonexistent.

A major cost advantage to Web-based surveys over print surveys is that the expenses of printing and folding the survey and of addressing, stuffing, and stamping envelopes are completely eliminated. Of course, these expenses are replaced with Web development costs that can be significant,[2] although these costs are one time expenses.

Multimedia elements can now be easily added to any survey in a Web environment. These elements can be in the question or in the response list. Full color images can be included in the survey and mouse clicks used to identify specific image locations that can be easily recorded and stored.

Web surveys allow for "skip" and "context" logic. An example in a paper survey is the type of question that says, "If you answer yes to question 5, skip to question 8." In an online situation the computer can automatically skip to question 8 without ever showing question 6 and 7.

Context logic allows the survey to modify itself based on a previous response. For example, if the person responding to the survey created by Slepski[7] indicates that he or she is a physician, question 4 is seen (**Fig. 1**). If the respondent indicates that he or she is a nurse, a different version of the question is seen (**Fig. 2**). The only difference is the choices of response based on the context of a previously answered question relating to their designated role.

When programming the survey, the questions can be embedded within an instructional application. There is no rule that says a survey must include a fixed number of items all placed on the same page or adjacent pages. One can include survey questions throughout an online instructional application.

There are three ways to implement a Web-based survey. The easiest way is to use an online Web service such as SurveyMonkey, QuestionPro, or Zoomerang. These services have free demo accounts one can use for small surveys; however, for anything of a reasonable scale, the "pay for" version is required so that one is not limited to the number of questions that can be asked or the number of people who can respond. One should check with his or her institution to see if they already have a site license or contract with one of these companies. The advantage of using a commercial Web service is there is absolutely no computer programming involved.

SurveyMonkey was used for the survey shown in **Fig. 3**. The questions are typed in much like in a simple word processor. Although one does not have as much control over the screen layout, the ease of developing a survey may more than compensate for that deficiency. The output will be to a Web table (that can be copy or pasted into Excel) or an Excel readable spreadsheet that can be downloaded to the desktop for further data analysis (**Fig. 4**).

In some online Web survey services, data can be saved directly to an SPSS (Statistical Package for the Social Sciences) format. Another benefit to using one of these types of services is that one is not responsible for maintaining software on a server. Unless technology people are closely available or the technical challenge is desired, one is not going to want to get into the software and hardware maintenance area. The big downside is the need to limit the survey to the formatting of the Web service. As long as their template works for the survey, this is fine; however, if one wants

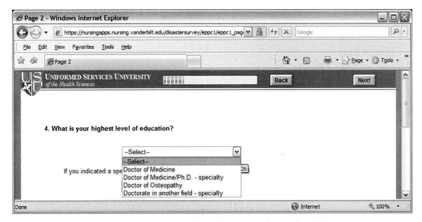

Fig. 1. Context sensitive dropdown choice for physicians from Slepski's survey.

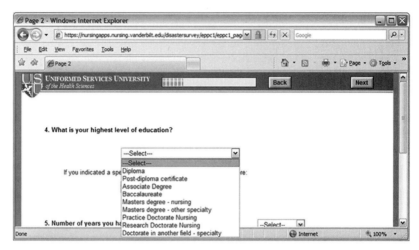

Fig. 2. Context sensitive dropdown choice for nurses from Slepski's survey.

special features such as multimedia objects placed in specific locations on the screen, wants the survey embedded inside of an instructional module, or wants multiple questions on single lines, these applications will not work.

A second approach is to purchase a "canned" survey tool and to mount it on a server that can be accessed and controlled. The primary advantage of this approach

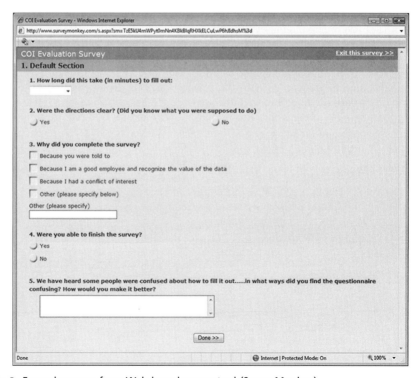

Fig. 3. Example screen from Web-based survey tool (SurveyMonkey).

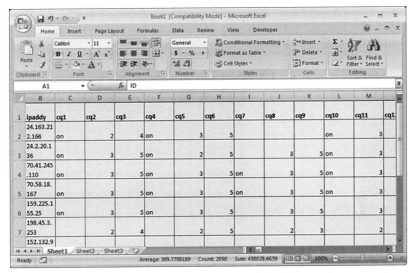

Fig. 4. Spreadsheet style output of survey responses. Each line is a set of responses from one person.

over the previous one is the avoidance of recurring "rental" costs. These tools work much like the commercial Web sites, but one must pay for the software up front once, after which it can continue to be used cost free for the life of the software license. Although some of the applications allow a bit more control over screen design, one is still limited to whatever they provide. Examples of this type of software are ClassApps, Prezza Checkbox, Apian SurveyPro, or SurveyGold.

For persons who are adventurous with technology, a personal survey software application can be created and mounted on a personal server. Although this can involve a substantial amount of work, initially, one has the benefits of completely controlling all aspects of the survey. One can decide how questions are to be displayed; one can introduce logic that presents different questions based on different answers to early questions (skip and context logic); one can introduce multimedia elements; and, if the survey is created in the same product used to create online instruction, one can embed the survey within an instructional module. The survey creator can decide what they want as output and how it is formatted, displayed, and distributed. In the survey shown in **Fig. 5**, there are three responses required for each assessment area.

The downside of this approach is the fact that programming is involved. Online surveys are composed of three elements, and one must create each of the three.[8] The first element is the front end Web site that displays the question. The second is the middleware that takes the data the respondent puts into the Web form objects on the Web page (eg, text boxes, checkboxes, radio buttons, dropdowns) and pushes it into the database application. The third is the back end which is the database itself. In addition, one must build a middleware utility that can extract the data out of the database and display it either on a Web page or in an Excel readable document to perform data analysis.

The front end can be developed with a Web editor such as GoLive, FrontPage, or Dreamweaver; however, some excellent Web development tools can provide added functionality. Lectora, from Trivantis, makes the programming of the front end much easier. It is fully drag and drop, reminiscent of PowerPoint. The great feature of Lectora

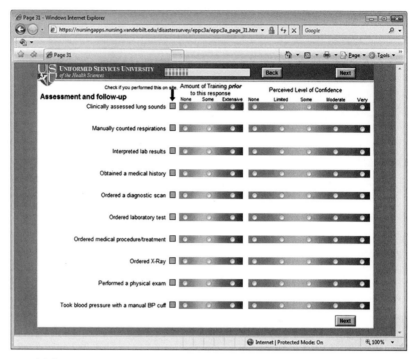

Fig. 5. Multiple questions per line require computer coding and currently cannot be done from "canned" Web products.

is the JavaScript title manager that stores variables and responses across multiple pages in the survey and outputs them at one time, upon pressing a Submit button, to the middleware program. Without such a feature, one must either submit the responses to the middleware after each page (making it difficult for the respondent to go back and change a response) or create a cookie code to store responses until the responses are submitted. Both approaches require significant programming skill; therefore, the use of the title manager is an excellent feature.

Several downsides to creating Web-based surveys can affect the number and quality of responses. First, there is the programming cost. Creating a survey, particularly from scratch, requires significant programming skills. One must be aware of the computer languages supported on the hosting server. Examples would be ASP (VBScript or server side JavaScript), ASP.NET, PHP, or Perl. If you do not have those skills and cannot acquire the services of someone with them, this approach is not for you.

Second, if the server is down, people cannot get to the survey, and most likely they will not come back. One should ensure that the environment the survey is placed on is stable with an extremely high uptime, or some of the sample will be lost.

Third, although research shows good response rates for online surveys, some audiences will not appear. If a person has weak or nonexistent network connectivity, they will not be heard from. Additionally, some people do not like reading from a screen and will not take the time to complete the survey if it is too long.

Fourth, a malicious person can flood the survey with multiple completion attempts. This activity can be recognized by recording the IP address of the machine they are using to complete the survey.

ISSUES TO CONSIDER WHEN CREATING A WEB-BASED SURVEY

One must be aware of probable screen resolutions the respondents will have. Today in 2008, it is reasonable to expect 1024 × 768 resolution. The survey should be created to account for that. If it is known that respondents do not have that resolution, one must adjust the survey accordingly. Users will put up with vertical scrolling as long as it is not a long screen. Horizontal scrolling is unacceptable because respondents will have to scroll right for each written line longer than the width of their screen and will give up after awhile. One should also keep in mind that the survey should be slightly smaller than the expected resolution to account for the size of the browser frame.

One should consider not numbering questions or assigning "a," "b," and "c" style subscripts to the numbers of skipped questions. Skipped questions always need to be on a screen of their own so they can be skipped over without the respondent seeing them. In a paper survey there is no problem with a skipped question because the respondent still gets to see it. Online if a respondent answers question 5 and the next question number seen is question 8, he or she may wonder what was missed because it was not seen. Smart users will figure out to answer question 5 differently to see the skipped questions; however, the respondent may never go back and correct the answer to question 5, giving bad data on that question. Alternately, instead of numbering questions 5, 6, 7, and 8, one should number them as 5, 5a, 5b, and then 6. If skipped, users will go immediately from question 5 to 6. If not skipped, respondents will go from 5 to 5a and 5b and then to 6. In either case, persons who skip questions will not be aware that they skipped anything.

The total number of questions should be kept to 256 or under. Although this may not seem like a real problem (who would create a survey with that many items), it is important to remember that every checkbox counts as its own question. For example, if a question asks, "Check all the meals you ate today" and lists four checkboxes (ie, breakfast, lunch, dinner, and snack), from a system perspective that translates to four separate questions out of the 256. With checkboxes, it is easy to approach that question limit. We recommend having no more than 256 items because, with that number, it is relatively simple to download the data into an Excel spreadsheet. Excel is currently limited to no more than 256 columns, which would allow the survey owner to put the entire dataset into a single spreadsheet for analysis purposes. If more than 256 questions are needed, one should try to lump them into no more than 256 item chunks. Some unique identifier (eg, a username or the exact time to the second the respondent starts the first part of the survey) will have to be created in each table, otherwise you will not be able to know which record corresponds to whom. The easiest solution is to stay within the 256-item limit which allows one to store everything in one Excel table. Shorter really is better, as long as the information needed is obtained. Surveys that take more than 15 minutes to complete are often abandoned before submission takes place.[9] Expecting respondents to sit in a stiff chair viewing a monitor for more than 30 minutes is asking a lot. With more than that time, response rates will be significantly lower.

One should always have a Forward/Next button and a Back button on each page in the survey to allow the respondent to go back and change an answer after thinking about it (**Fig. 6**). No responses should be submitted to the database until the survey is complete. If the survey allows a respondent to submit on each page, it makes it difficult to allow him or her to go back and change an item without having both responses recorded in the database. One should ensure that the Submit button looks different from or is in a different location than the Next button to clue the respondent that

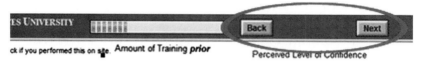

Fig. 6. Clearly defined navigation buttons in the survey make completion much easier.

something different is about to happen and to pay attention. Once the person submits responses, every effort should be made to keep him or her from going back and changing responses, otherwise it is likely that multiple submissions will occur from the same person (**Fig. 7**).

A thank you page should always appear at the end of the survey.[4] This page needs to show up after the final Submit button has been pressed at the end. This page serves two purposes. First, it politely thanks the person for participating and provides any additional information, such as where one can see the results, or directions to close all copies of browsers. Second, and most importantly, it gets the respondent off of the page with the Submit button. The problem that occurs if respondents stay on the page with the Submit button is that they are never sure whether their data was submitted; therefore, they click the Submit button again, and again, and again, polluting the database with duplicate records that are difficult to purge (**Fig. 8**).

A progress bar or progress notification system should be included at the top of each page in the survey. People like to know how far along they are in the survey and how much more they have to do. On paper, that is easy by simply looking at the number of pages, whereas online it is difficult because the respondent only sees the page they are on. The last thing you want is for someone to get within one page of completing the survey, only to give up before submission because they do not know how much longer they have (**Fig. 9**).

One should always record the IP address, the date (based on the server clock), and the time the survey starts (to the second and also based on the server clock) when possible. Although it is not an absolute indicator, if the same survey is filled out a dozen times with the same IP address, one may have cause to be suspicious that the same person is filling out the survey multiple times. Nevertheless, there are some legitimate reasons why the same IP may show up multiple times. For example, Slepski[7] recently

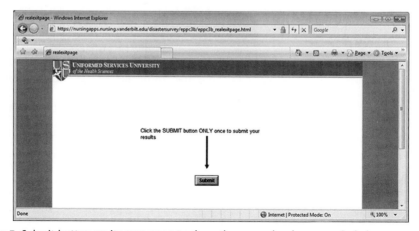

Fig. 7. Submit button on its own page to show the survey has been concluded.

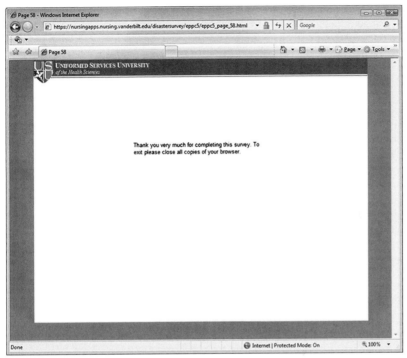

Fig. 8. Getting users off the Submit button page keeps them from polluting the dataset by clicking submit over and over.

created a survey for Katrina disaster responders and found several husband and wife teams responding to Katrina and answering the survey from the same computer. Another situation in which that may occur is in the workplace. Through a networking configuration, respondents may share an externally reported IP address. Multiple entries with the same IP are not an absolute indicator of a problem but will give you data to consider.

The date and time are critical to record for several reasons. First, most responses can be expected to occur within about 36 hours[9] after people are made aware of the survey's Web address. If people report that they can not get on and many respondents are seen around that time, one can be fairly sure that the problem is either a network traffic jam or the result of the server getting overloaded with traffic. In that case one may wish to spread out who receives survey information by reducing the numbers of people who know about at the same time. One should also record the time the

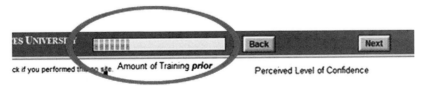

Fig. 9. A progress bar gives the person a clue as to how far they have gone and how much more they have to do. It reduces the likelihood of abandoning the survey early.

Submit button is clicked. The difference will give the duration it took to complete the survey. The survey may need to be shortened if it takes too long. Another reason for recording the time is the opportunity to look for "breaks" in the times people fill the survey out. Some of the breaks may be explainable (eg, no night time submissions if the survey only covers people in adjacent time zones), whereas large unexplained gaps may indicate a network, survey, or software problem that is preventing people from responding. One should look for patterns when this occurs and try to get in around those times to determine if there is a problem.

If an e-mail is sent out with the Web address of the survey, the Web address should be placed on its own line in the e-mail and the Enter key pressed to insert a blank line after the address. That action turns the address into a hyperlink on which the user can simply click to get to the survey. If a hyperlink is not provided, the user will have to copy/paste the link into a Web browser or type it in from scratch. Either approach is more difficult and will cut the survey response rate.

One should know who will respond, the power of the machines they will likely respond on, and their network connectivity. If they are using weaker machines or have narrower band network connectivity, multimedia elements should be kept to a minimum. People will not wait around for a Flash movie to load and display. If most of the respondents have bandwidth issues, graphics should be limited as well.[4]

One should be creative in constructing a survey. A survey could be embedded throughout a computer-assisted instruction Web application. If the respondents will have strong machines with strong network connectivity, graphics and animations can be combined to make the survey more interesting. The more interesting the survey is, the greater the likelihood it will be completed.

The survey should be checked on multiple browsers. What looks good in Internet Explorer may not format correctly in Firefox and vice versa. If JavaScript must be enabled or if any special players are needed, such as Flash player, respondents should know in advance. One should check what is seen if respondents do not have the correct player or functionality enabled.

One should use only Web-safe fonts and avoid fonts named after cities. The site should be checked on multiple copies of the browser on different machines to see how the fonts display. Use of narrowly available fonts may result in screens that are difficult to read as the browser tries to map to an acceptable alternative font. Our experience is that fonts the browser thinks may be an acceptable alternative may not be acceptable to you. The font should be kept consistent (no change from page to page) and the number of different fonts on a page kept to a minimum to avoid a "ransom note" look. Sans serif fonts look cleaner and are easier to read but allow people to become confused between zeros and "O's" and ones and "L's." If identifying and distinguishing between these entities is significant in the survey, a serif font should be used.

The dropdown choice is an excellent example of something that will give data comparable to a radio button but uses a lot less screen geography; however, one should ensure that a "—Select—" choice is the first choice showing in the dropdown. If the first choice showing is a legitimate choice and the respondent really meant to skip that question, that first choice is reported as their choice even though that was not intended (eg, too many people in surveys report living in Alabama). If uncertainty remains as to whether all of the reasonable choices have been included in a dropdown (or checkbox set), an "Other" option should be included along with a free text area for "Please specify." The pilot data should then be examined to determine whether more options should be added. In the dropdown displayed in **Fig. 10**, there is a "—Select—" choice first and "Other" choice at the bottom, with a textbox (hidden from view) for respondents to fill out more detail if they select "Other."

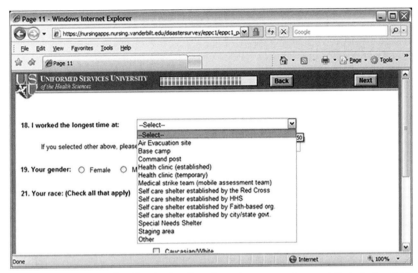

Fig. 10. Creating a bogus first line in the dropdown box prevents a real first choice that was unselected from being reported to the database as selected.

The survey owner should never be able to access the actual database on the server live and in real time. There is too much risk that the database could be damaged or locked, preventing others from responding at that time. One should either download the database regularly to a local machine and examine it there, or create a "view" that will allow the survey owner to see the data in a Web table or as a download into an Excel readable file (either XLS or CSV). The Web address to access the entire dataset in an HTML table should be a secret and unlinked to any other Web page to prevent a Google or Yahoo spider from finding the page and reporting it in a Web search. To protect the security of the data, there must be no way to change the data as well as safeguards to ensure that only appropriate people can see the data. Rules from the Health Insurance Portability and Accountability Act (HIPAA) and the Family Educational Rights and Privacy Act (FERPA) may apply.

For data of a sensitive nature, the survey should be hosted on an HTTPS Secure Sockets Level (SSL) server rather than a server without SSL. A server without SSL will display just HTTP in the URL line, not HTTPS. SSL encrypts the data so that if someone on the network is "packet sniffing" they will not see the actual responses but what appears to be a random collection of letters, symbols, and numbers. This idea is particularly important if the survey requires users to log in with usernames and passwords for security reasons.

Some people are not adept at using a mouse; therefore, the tab order corresponding to the sequence the questions appear on the page should be kept to allow the respondent to tab to the next question rather than mouse over to it.

The survey should be consistent in where navigation buttons are placed, what they look like, and how they behave. Although we strongly recommend placing Next buttons at the top of the page and at the bottom, you may only want them at the bottom to force the respondent to get there. If they are at the top, they should be positioned consistently on each page rather than appearing to jump around from page to page. When the respondent reaches the Submit button at the end, it should have its own distinctive look, and the respondent should be warned that pressing that button submits their data. Next and Back buttons must account for any skip logic, as mentioned earlier.

Popups or downloads should be avoided in the survey. Many browsers are default configured to block these entities. Often, popups, even if they are displayed, appear behind the survey's window and are eclipsed by the survey. Unless the respondent is particularly technically savvy, they may never see the popup.

One should decide how many people will be responding to the survey at one time, that is, how many will be pressing the Submit button within seconds of each other. Microsoft Access is metered to allow up to about five people to submit at once. If more concurrency is expected, concern about file lock will result in more than five timing out. Respondents will spend time completing the survey, only to get to the end and not be able to submit. If five concurrent submissions are too low a threshold, the survey should be migrated over to a more powerful database engine such as Microsoft SQL, Oracle, or MySQL.

Because open-ended questions are more complex to analyze,[5] one may want to rewrite questions into a closed-ended format. For example, if the respondent is asked to put in their weight, he or she may enter "120," "120 lbs," or "120 pounds." Internally, these answers are not the same. On the other hand, if a dropdown had numbers between 90 and 240 that a person selected, the data would be more easy to analyze, avoiding the need to remove, at the programming level, the extra verbiage in the response. The programmer writing the script that connects the HTML front end to the database must remember to remove apostrophes from student free text responses. Apostrophes in responses break the SQL queries in the middleware scripts and cause the data to not go into the database.

The survey should be consistent in answer choices. If Yes/No questions are asked, "Yes" and "No" should be placed in the same order for all of those questions. If missing data is coded as 99, it should be so for every question.

An attempt should be made to keep the Web address simple. If that is difficult, one should create a simple Web address on a server that can be accessed and then put a redirector or 100% width frameset pointer to the "real" location. In that way, if the survey passes word of mouth, users will not have a long URL to type in.

A question item numbering or naming schema should be developed that makes sense. For example, mnemonic names could be used for Web form fields. One should use whatever names are selected for the form field names as the names of the variables the programmer uses in the middleware program. Those same names should also be used as the column names in the database. In that way, if something does not show up in the database, it is easier to follow the trail back to the Web file. One should avoid names that are reserved words, such as "date." Instead, use something like "todaysdate."

One should avoid data normalization (placing data from one record in multiple tables) and store each record in a single table in the database to make it easier later to download the data into either SPSS or Excel.

One should avoid multiple framed windows and text stored as a graphic rather than text. Screen readers for the site impaired cannot interpret graphically stored text and have trouble analyzing frames. A 508 compliance is a requirement for products contracted for the US Federal Government.

The survey should be tested out with a small group of field testers to examine every option and every branch. In that way, one can detect any problems with the logic, question wording, multimedia components, and basic design before the survey is sent out to large numbers of potential respondents.[10]

THE PERSONAL DIGITAL ASSISTANT AS A DATA COLLECTION TOOL

PDAs (eg, a Palm or Windows Mobile device) can be used to collect data in the field. Typically, the scenario is the researcher goes out to the data collection site and inputs data into the PDA, brings the PDA back at a later time, and synchs it to their computer. The file then gets uploaded and integrated into an existing database on a server. At the authors' center, nursing students collect clinical encounter data on their PDAs and upload it to the server weekly so that their preceptors and faculty can see what they have been doing for the week. This approach eliminates the need for the student to record the data twice, once on paper at the bedside and again that evening on the Web. With the PDA they record it only once, at bedside, and then synch and upload. We developed the PDA side of our student assigned Patient Encounter Clinical log[11] at the direct request of our students who wanted to simplify their data collection process.

There are limitations and issues associated with PDA use for data collection. First, there is a limited screen size called "screen geography." A single screen on a Web site will take multiple screens on a PDA (**Fig. 11**), and one cannot organize the questions on the screen with the same flexibility as when using a Web interface.

One must decide early on which operating system will be supported. At the time of this writing, there are four widely used personal handheld operating systems (eg, Windows Mobile, Palm, Symbian, and Blackberry). If all four systems will be supported, you have to find a database application that is operating system agnostic yet within your budget.

PDAs are prone to data errors. They are not computers. There is insufficient development space to create a lot of error checking capability. On occasion, the authors have noticed that entire data fields do not transfer when synched. The entire synching and upload processes are a bit arcane and require some technology capabilities on the part of the user. Upload utilities to a database either need to be created or acquired.

Because of the portable nature of PDAs, if they are lost or stolen, any data not already transferred is also lost or stolen. If that data contains confidential information, the loss could present a HIPAA violation or worse.

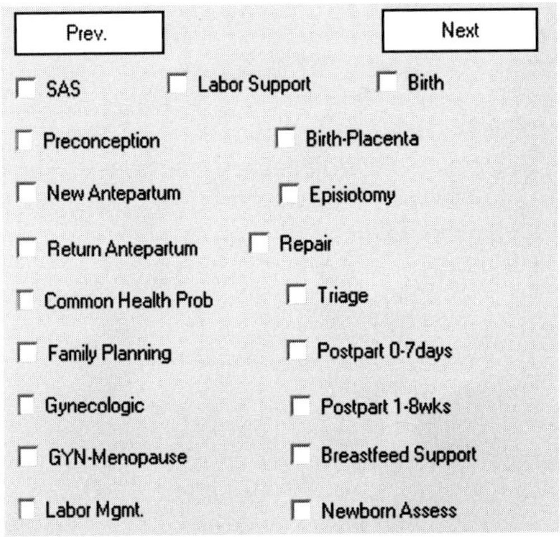

Fig. 11. PDA screens limit screen geography but are useful data entry alternatives to a standard personal computer–based Web page.

PDA data collection can be a viable approach for data collection if you can control who is going o use it and what operating system they are going to use, and if you have the ability to test and write programs that will assimilate the data into a database application.

SUMMARY

The Internet and its attending technologies provide an excellent platform for researchers to collect data. The combination of e-mail, the Web, and PDAs covers the range of tools one needs to actively collect data relatively inexpensively over a large geographic area. The Web provides acceptable degrees of anonymity while making reasonably certain that a survey is not getting overwhelmed by one person replying over and over. The ability to implement logic in a survey as well as include multimedia elements takes survey administration to the next level and is far better than traditional paper and pencil approaches that can use neither. The ability to have data go directly into a database not only speeds up the possibilities for data analysis but also virtually eliminates transcription errors caused by carelessness or the inability to read handwriting. E-mail technology makes it easy to send even the most complex Web address to a wide range of users. PDA technology allows the researcher to collect data in the field using a highly portable pocket-sized device. The downsides to these approaches are that the software development and maintenance side is not inexpensive, multimedia elements may require viewers (such as Flash player) that may not be on everyone's machine, and not everyone in a potential population has Internet access. Nevertheless, the costs are decreasing, particularly for Web service products. Products that view multimedia are becoming fairly standardized, and today most people have some type of Internet access, even if it is through a centralized location such as a school or library.

REFERENCES

1. Roberts LD. Opportunities and constraints of electronic research. In: Reynolds RA, Woods R, Baker JD, editors. Handbook of research on electronic surveys and measurements. Hershey (PA): Idea Group; 2007. p. 19–27.
2. Jansen KJ, Corley KG, Jansen BJ. E-survey methodology. In: Reynolds RA, Woods R, Baker JD, editors. Handbook of research on electronic surveys and measurements. Hershey (PA): Idea Group; 2007. p. 1–8.
3. Sing J, Burgess S. Electronic data collection methods. In: Reynolds RA, Woods R, Baker JD, editors. Handbook of research on electronic surveys and measurements. Hershey (PA): Idea Group; 2007. p. 28–43.
4. Lumsden J. Online questionnaire design guidelines. In: Reynolds RA, Woods R, Baker JD, editors. Handbook of research on electronic surveys and measurements. Hershey (PA): Idea Group; 2007. p. 44–64.
5. Sue MV, Ritter LA. Conducting online surveys. Thousand Oaks (CA): Sage Publications; 2007.
6. Dixon R, Turner R. Electronic vs. conventional surveys. In: Reynolds RA, Woods R, Baker JD, editors. Handbook of research on electronic surveys and measurements. Hershey (PA): Idea Group; 2007. p. 104–11.
7. Slepski L. Emergency preparedness and professional competency among health care providers during hurricanes Katrina and Rita survey. Bethesda (MD): Uniformed Services University of the Health Sciences; 2007.

8. Artz JM. Software design tips for online surveys. In: Reynolds RA, Woods R, Baker JD, editors. Handbook of research on electronic surveys and measurements. Hershey (PA): Idea Group; 2007. p. 76–82.

9. Amplitude Research. Online surveys: best practices for customer and employee feedback (white paper). 2003. Available at: www.amplitude.com/white.shtml. Accessed November, 2007.

10. Iarossi G. The power of survey design. Washington (DC): The World Bank; 2006.

11. McNew R. Online clinical log (software). Nashville (TN): Vanderbilt University; 2005.

Index

Note: Page numbers of article titles are in **boldface** type.

C

Clinical information system, faculty development initiatives for integration into nursing education, 526–530

Clinical nursing education, Web-based, tools for, 543–544

Collaboration tools, for Web-based nursing education, 539

Communication tools, for Web-based nursing education, 539

Community of learning model, in online education for doctoral nursing programs, 559–561

Competencies, in technology and informatics, **507–521**
  forces driving preparation in informatics, 511–513
  health care information technologies, 508–511
  master list of, for nurses, 513–519

Computer skills, guidance with, for online learning, 551

Content development, tools for Web-based nursing education, 542–543

Course management systems, for Web-based nursing education, 536–538

Critical thinking, simulation technology in nursing education, **593–603**

Culturally competent care, online transcultural nursing courses and, **567–574**

Curriculum, nursing, for online transcultural nursing courses, **567–574**

D

Distance education. *See also* Online learning.
  in doctoral nursing programs, **557–566**
    challenges in, 562–564
    community of inquiry model, 559–561
    evaluation, 564–565
    initial efforts in, 558–559
    technologies to support, 561–562
  supporting integration of into nursing education, **497–506**

Diversity, challenges of, 567–568
  responses to, 568
  transcultural nursing courses online, **567–574**

Doctoral programs, nursing, distance education in, **557–566**
  challenges in, 562–564
  community of inquiry model, 559–561
  evaluation, 564–565
  initial efforts in, 558–559
  technologies to support, 561–562

E

E-mail, survey data collection via, 605–606

Education, nursing, technology in, 497–609
  doctoral programs, distance education in, **557–566**
    challenges in, 562–564

Nurs Clin N Am 43 (2008) 621–627
doi:10.1016/S0029-6465(08)00069-8
0029-6465/08/$ – see front matter
nursing.theclinics.com

Moving?

Make sure your subscription moves with you!

To notify us of your new address, find your **Clinics Account Number** (located on your mailing label above your name), and contact customer service at:

E-mail: elspcs@elsevier.com

800-654-2452 (subscribers in the U.S. & Canada)
1-407-563-6020 (subscribers outside of the U.S. & Canada)

Fax number: 407-363-9661

Elsevier Periodicals Customer Service
6277 Sea Harbor Drive
Orlando, FL 32887-4800

*To ensure uninterrupted delivery of your subscription, please notify us at least 4 weeks in advance of move.

United States Postal Service

Statement of Ownership, Management, and Circulation
(All Periodicals Publications Except Requestor Publications)

1. Publication Title	2. Publication Number	3. Filing Date
Nursing Clinics of North America	5 9 8 - 9 6 0	9/15/08

4. Issue Frequency	5. Number of Issues Published Annually	6. Annual Subscription Price
Mar, Jun, Sep, Dec	4	$123.00

7. Complete Mailing Address of Known Office of Publication (Not printer) (Street, city, county, state, and ZIP+4)

Elsevier Inc.
360 Park Avenue South
New York, NY 10010-1710

Contact Person
Stephen Bushing
Telephone (Include area code)
215-239-3688

8. Complete Mailing Address of Headquarters or General Business Office of Publisher (Not printer)

Elsevier Inc., 360 Park Avenue South, New York, NY 10010-1710

9. Full Names and Complete Mailing Addresses of Publisher, Editor, and Managing Editor (Do not leave blank)

Publisher (Name and complete mailing address)

John Schrefer, Elsevier, Inc., 1600 John F. Kennedy Blvd. Suite 1800, Philadelphia, PA 19103-2899

Editor (Name and complete mailing address)

Alexandra Gavenda, Elsevier, Inc., 1600 John F. Kennedy Blvd. Suite 1800, Philadelphia, PA 19103-2899

Managing Editor (Name and complete mailing address)

Catherine Bewick, Elsevier, Inc., 1600 John F. Kennedy Blvd. Suite 1800, Philadelphia, PA 19103-2899

10. Owner (Do not leave blank. If the publication is owned by a corporation, give the name and address of the corporation immediately followed by the names and addresses of all stockholders owning or holding 1 percent or more of the total amount of stock. If not owned by a corporation, give the names and addresses of the individual owners. If owned by a partnership or other unincorporated firm, give its name and address as well as those of each individual owner. If the publication is published by a nonprofit organization, give its name and address.)

Full Name	Complete Mailing Address
Wholly owned subsidiary of	4520 East-West Highway
Reed/Elsevier, US holdings	Bethesda, MD 20814

11. Known Bondholders, Mortgagees, and Other Security Holders Owning or Holding 1 Percent or More of Total Amount of Bonds, Mortgages, or Other Securities. If none, check box ☐ None

Full Name	Complete Mailing Address
N/A	

12. Tax Status (For completion by nonprofit organizations authorized to mail at nonprofit rates) (Check one)
The purpose, function, and nonprofit status of this organization and the exempt status for federal income tax purposes:
☐ Has Not Changed During Preceding 12 Months
☐ Has Changed During Preceding 12 Months (Publisher must submit explanation of change with this statement)

PS Form 3526, September 2006 (Page 1 of 3 (Instructions Page 3)) PSN 7530-01-000-9931 PRIVACY NOTICE: See our Privacy policy in www.usps.com

---

13. Publication Title		14. Issue Date for Circulation Data Below
Nursing Clinics of North America		September 2008

15. Extent and Nature of Circulation		Average No. Copies Each Issue During Preceding 12 Months	No. Copies of Single Issue Published Nearest to Filing Date
a. Total Number of Copies (Net press run)		3475	3400
b. Paid Circulation (By Mail and Outside the Mail)	(1) Mailed Outside-County Paid Subscriptions Stated on PS Form 3541. (Include paid distribution above nominal rate, advertiser's proof copies, and exchange copies)	2068	1978
	(2) Mailed In-County Paid Subscriptions Stated on PS Form 3541 (Include paid distribution above nominal rate, advertiser's proof copies, and exchange copies)		
	(3) Paid Distribution Outside the Mails Including Sales Through Dealers and Carriers, Street Vendors, Counter Sales, and Other Paid Distribution Outside USPS®	525	570
	(4) Paid Distribution by Other Classes Mailed Through the USPS (e.g. First-Class Mail®)		
c. Total Paid Distribution (Sum of 15b (1), (2), (3), and (4))		2593	2548
d. Free or Nominal Rate Distribution (By Mail and Outside the Mail)	(1) Free or Nominal Rate Outside-County Copies Included on PS Form 3541	51	70
	(2) Free or Nominal Rate In-County Copies Included on PS Form 3541		
	(3) Free or Nominal Rate Copies Mailed at Other Classes Mailed Through the USPS (e.g. First-Class Mail)		
	(4) Free or Nominal Rate Distribution Outside the Mail (Carriers or other means)		
e. Total Free or Nominal Rate Distribution (Sum of 15d (1), (2), (3) and (4))		51	70
f. Total Distribution (Sum of 15c and 15e)		2644	2618
g. Copies not Distributed (See instructions to publishers #4 (page #3))		831	782
h. Total (Sum of 15f and g)		3475	3400
i. Percent Paid (15c divided by 15f times 100)		98.07%	97.33%

16. Publication of Statement of Ownership

☐ If the publication is a general publication, publication of this statement is required. Will be printed in the December 2008 issue of this publication.   ☐ Publication not required

17. Signature and Title of Editor, Publisher, Business Manager, or Owner	Date
(signature) Stephen R. Bushing – Executive Director of Subscription Services	September 15, 2008

I certify that all information furnished on this form is true and complete. I understand that anyone who furnishes false or misleading information on this form or who omits material or information requested on the form may be subject to criminal sanctions (including fines and imprisonment) and/or civil sanctions (including civil penalties).

PS Form 3526, September 2006 (Page 2 of 3)